D0193291

EVERYTHING
YOU NEED TO KNOW ABOUT...
Pregnancy

EVERYTHING

YOU NEED TO KNOW ABOUT...

Pregnancy

PAULA FORD-MARTIN

WITH ELISABETH A. ARON, M.D., F.A.C.O.G.

David & Charles

A DAVID & CHARLES BOOK

David & Charles is a subsidiary of F&W (UK) Ltd.,
an F&W Publications Inc. company

First published in the UK in 2004
First published in the USA as The Everything® Pregnancy Book,
by Adams Media Corporation in 2002

Project Manager Ian Kearey
Cover Design Ali Myer

A catalogue record for this book is available from the British Library.

ISBN 0 7153 1959 0

Printed in Great Britain by CPI Bath
for David & Charles
Brunel House   Newton Abbot   Devon

Visit our website at www.davidandcharles.co.uk

David & Charles books are available from all good bookshops;
alternatively you can contact our Orderline on (0)1626 334555 or
write to us at FREEPOST EX2110, David & Charles Direct,
Newton Abbot, TQ12 4ZZ (no stamp required UK mainland).

Contents

Acknowledgments

A special thank you to Dr Elisabeth Aron for lending her perspective and expertise to this book, and to Barb Doyen and Eric M. Hall for their patience, encouragement and guidance.

I'd also like to acknowledge the contributions and assistance of those women who offered their professional expertise and guidance to the writing of this book, including: Robin Elise Weiss, BA, LCCE, ICCE-CPE, CD (DONA) – woman of many acronyms, mother of five, and birthing partner extraordinaire – who was kind enough to share her wisdom; Dr Melissa Stöppler, whose stress management advice was invaluable on a personal as well as a professional level; and patient advocate and bestselling author Mary Shomon, who was a wealth of information on postpartum thyroid issues.

Top Ten Things
Every Pregnant Woman Should Know

1. Morning sickness doesn't just happen in the morning.

2. Alcohol and tobacco in any amount in pregnancy can have serious health repercussions for your baby.

3. Taking 400 micrograms of folic acid before and in early pregnancy can dramatically reduce your risk of having a baby with neural tube defects.

4. Trust your instincts – what worked for your neighbour, friend or sister isn't necessarily what's right for you.

5. A birth plan can help you and your partner work towards the labour and delivery experience you want.

6. Things don't always go according to plan, but being prepared for the possibilities can make the detours easier to handle.

7. A due date is a suggestion, not a contractual obligation.

8. Career and family are not mutually exclusive.

9. Legislation provides specific protections against pregnancy discrimination in the workplace.

10. Stress can be hard on the health of you and your baby; make sure you have a support system for both pregnancy and new motherhood.

Introduction

▶YOUR MOTHER ALWAYS SAID, 'You'll understand when you have kids of your own.' And as much as you may hate to admit it, she's right. Being a mum starts the day you find out you're no longer a solo act; suddenly responsibility means more than remembering when the cat needs an injection and getting the oil in the car changed every 3,000 miles. Pregnancy initiates you into an empathetic sisterhood of women who can be a source of inspiration, support and advice throughout pregnancy and beyond.

It's a big club, but it's surprisingly intimate in its knowledge of the trials and tribulations of motherhood. Never again will you roll your eyes at a toddler throwing a tantrum in the supermarket, or tap your fingers impatiently at that woman taking forever to load up her kids in the car and pull out of 'your' parking space. Mothers understand that pregnancy and parenting take a lot of patience, love and compassion.

Pregnancy also means preparing for a whole new lifestyle. You and your partner will no longer be couples-only; your free time will focus on parks and playgroups rather than dinner and a film. If you have children already, the challenges and joys of new sibling relationships are ahead. And your husband or partner will be exploring his new role as a dad and learning the ropes of child care. It's an exciting time, but as with any unfamiliar venture, pregnancy and the prospect of this completely dependent tiny person can inspire anxiety and, yes, even fear. Are you eating the right foods? Is your morning run bad for your baby? Will your child develop your grandfather's diabetes? In true motherly style, you've started worrying about your baby's well-being already.

Of course, your health-care team is the best source of information for specific medical questions about your pregnancy. But even the most dedicated doctor can't be at your disposal 24-7. This book was designed as your personal pregnancy assistant – an essential educational reference for your pregnancy concerns and a guide for the more practical matters of career considerations, car seats and family budgets. It's also a great resource for helping you plan a birth experience you'll treasure.

Most important, this book encourages open dialogue with your health-care team. Your doctor or midwife can provide medical care and expert advice, but ultimately you must manage your health care for yourself. That means reading, asking questions and making sure you're satisfied with the answers. After all, you wouldn't let your financial planner do whatever he pleases with your money without providing some input and approval. Yet many women don't feel they have a right to 'bother' their doctors with their questions about a much more precious investment – their child.

You'll make many critical decisions throughout your pregnancy, from pursuing diagnostic testing and genetic counselling to your labour and delivery preferences. Educating yourself allows you to make informed choices and to make the most of your time with your doctor or midwife. Most health-care providers are more than willing to answer your questions; patients who do their homework demonstrate their commitment to a healthy pregnancy and make everyone's job easier in the long run. But remember, communication is key. Your questions *will* go unanswered if you fail to ask them.

Enjoy this special time, and consider this book a key part of your support team. That highly coveted 'mother's intuition' is usually made, not born, and will come in time as you become better acquainted with your growing baby and learn more about this exciting journey called pregnancy and parenthood.

Chapter 1

Getting Ready

Pregnancy is a time of big changes for your family, your body and your emotional equilibrium. Finding balance and keeping yourself healthy are crucial to creating the best possible environment for baby, both in and out of the womb.

So You're Pregnant...

You just found out you're pregnant. Perhaps you've been trying for just a few months, or maybe for a few years. There's also a good chance this baby has taken you by surprise. Planned or unplanned, pregnancy stirs up a wide spectrum of emotions. You may be on cloud nine and picking out nursery wallpaper patterns, or you may be in a state of shock, wondering how you're going to handle it all.

Relax. You're normal. Everyone reacts to the joys and jeopardies of pregnancy differently. Preparing yourself for the road ahead is the best way to overcome your fears and get a realistic picture of what pregnancy and motherhood are made of. So ask questions, read, take classes and talk to friends and family who have been there. There's no such thing as too much information when it comes to your (and your baby's) health.

A Different Kind of Family Tree

Even if you and your partner are the models of perfect health, you may have a history of chronic illness or medical disorders further back in your lineage that could have an impact on the health of your unborn child. Your doctor will ask you questions about your ethnic and racial heritage and family background (and that of the baby's father) to screen for medical conditions your child may be at risk for. Having the most complete and accurate information possible will help her determine what screening tests, if any, you may wish to consider.

If you uncover a history of medical problems in your family you were unaware of, keep in mind that only a tiny percentage of infants are born with a birth defect, and only a portion of those are thought to have a genetic component. In many cases of inherited diseases, a complex interaction of both genetic and environmental factors is required to trigger the condition. If your doctor decides you are at risk for passing along a medical problem to your child, she may refer you to a genetic counsellor for further analysis of your risk factors and a discussion of options for additional testing or another appropriate course of action.

Antentatal Visits

Even if you have a perfect pregnancy, you will be seeing a lot of your health-care provider over the next nine months. Once you have seen your GP and had the pregnancy confirmed, you will be called for a number of routine check-ups. How often you see health professionals and who you see varies between health authorities and individual pregnancies, but this is a basic guide.

Booking Appointment

The first, and longest, of the routine check-ups is known as the 'booking' appointment, which occurs between the eighth and twelfth weeks of pregnancy. Usually you will see a midwife at your local hospital, but if there are potential complications, such as a history of pregnancy problems or an existing chronic condition, you may also see the consultant obstetrician. If you are being cared for through a Domino system, your midwife will probably visit you at home.

If you are offered a home visit, it is worth considering, as your home environment is probably much more relaxing than the hospital, and if you have other children it is more convenient. This visit takes about an hour and a half. The midwife will need to take a detailed medical history and perform some routine tests. It helps to check with relatives (including your partner's) about any inherited conditions, so that you have this information to hand. You will also need to tell the midwife the average length of your menstrual cycles and the date of your last period. It's also a good idea to read any information your GP gave you and to note down any questions you have. Many women like their partner to attend this first appointment – it's a great way to feel involved with the new baby.

As well as all the paperwork, you will also be given a physical examination. This includes height and weight and blood pressure, and a sample of urine will be checked for glucose (which may indicate gestational diabetes) and protein (a possible sign of pre-eclampsia). You caregiver will also feel how your uterus is growing and may give you an internal examination. In some areas you may also be offered an early ultrasound at this visit. You will be given a copy of your notes, which you should bring to all your appointments.

Subsequent Appointments

The frequency of these varies, but you will probably see your caregiver about once a month. These check-ups are much shorter than the booking appointment and involve a weight, urine and blood pressure check. Your caregiver will also check how the baby is growing.

Types of Antenatal Care

What type of care is available to you will depend on your health and risk factors, and also what is available in your area. Do speak to your caregivers early on about the types of care you will receive – midwife-led care is often available on a first-come-first-served basis, and facilities such as birthing centres can get booked up very quickly.

Shared Care

Most pregnancies handled by the NHS share your care between your GP and a team of midwives. You will attend the hospital for ultrasounds and any other tests, but generally see your own GP or midwife for routine check-ups. If the need arises, you will be referred to a consultant. Remember that GPs rarely get involved in the actual delivery.

Consultant Care

This type of care is usually offered to a women with a history of pregnancy problems, or who, for whatever reason, is considered high-risk. This means you will have all your appointments at the hospital and will see the consultant frequently, although hospital midwives will still carry out your routine tests.

Midwife-Led Care

As the name suggests, your midwife will be your primary caregiver, and you will see one of the team of midwives at home for most of your check-ups. If you are hoping for a home delivery, this will give you a chance to build a relationship with the midwife who will deliver your baby and care for you afterwards. Due to the shortage of midwives throughout the

NHS, this sort of care is not always available to everyone who would like to have it.

You can also employ the services of an independent midwife, and this is a popular option with women hoping for a home birth.

Domino system

In this type of care you work with the same group of midwives throughout your pregnancy and delivery (whether in hospital or at home), who will then visit you after the birth. You will have most of your appointments in your own home. Again, this type of care is not always available in all areas.

REMEMBER!

Don't be afraid to ask questions. It's easy to get swept along by the system, especially when staff are so busy. But this is your pregnancy and it is important that you feel informed and in control. It's a good idea to jot down your concerns and questions before you see your caregivers, as it's easy to forget with so much going on.

Thinking About the Birth

It may seem very early to be thinking about the delivery in great detail (in fact, you may be trying not to think about it!), but it's vital to think about your options as soon as possible. In an ideal world, every woman would be offered whatever type of care she wanted, but of course the reality is often very different. If you would like a home birth, you need to discuss this with your caregivers as soon as possible. By law every woman has the right to have a midwife attend her at home if there are no medical contraindications, but many health authorities just do not have enough staff. Additionally, your doctor may not be that keen on home births, or you may not be a suitable candidate. Whatever type of birth you are hoping for, talk your options through as soon as you can. Hospital procedures can vary dramatically. This is the time to ask about delivery-room protocol and facilities, not when your waters break.

Stopping Smoking

The life inside you is dependent on your 'delivery system' for its very existence. Taking care of yourself – body and mind – over these next nine months will be your number one priority for raising a healthy baby.

You don't need anyone to tell you that cigarettes are bad for you. If you are a smoker, you've probably tried to stop, possibly more than once. It's not easy, but now you have special motivation to stop and make it stick. In addition to the health risks smoking exposes you to, such as cardiovascular disease, lung cancer and high blood pressure, it can also have dire consequences for your baby.

When you smoke, the amount of oxygen in your bloodstream is reduced, and so is the oxygen supply to your baby. Babies born to smokers (either parent) are more likely to miscarry, be born prematurely or be of low birth weight. They are also at an increased risk of Sudden Infant Death Syndrome or Cot Death. Studies show that women are far more likely to stop smoking during pregnancy if their partner is not smoking either – so tell him that standing outside the back door for a quick cigarette is not enough. If necessary, ask your doctor for help to give up.

Studies have shown that women metabolize nicotine faster in pregnancy, meaning that you may actually require a larger dose of nicotine replacement therapy (NRT) than you would if you weren't pregnant. For this reason, your doctor should oversee the use of any NRT product to ensure its efficacy.

If you're a smoker, ideally you will kick the habit in the planning stages of your pregnancy. However, the good news is that even if you're pregnant and still smoking, stopping now can make a big difference to your baby's health. Women who stop smoking in the first trimester of pregnancy greatly reduce the risk of IUGR (inter-uterine growth restriction) for their child. For women who have difficulty stopping through conventional means, nicotine replacement therapies – in the form of gum, patches or inhalers – may be an option. Although these products are now available without a prescription, make sure you tell your doctor that you are considering using them. Be aware that the safety and effectiveness of NRT in pregnancy has not been extensively tested, and animal studies have indicated that nicotine exposure in the womb may cause later breathing problems in offspring. However, for the mother-to-be who smokes heavily and is not able to stop through traditional methods, their use is preferable to cigarettes, since they do not contain carbon monoxide or any of the other hundreds of toxic chemicals contained in cigarette smoke.

Street drugs

There is evidence that street drugs, such as cannabis, cross the placenta. This means that they enter the baby's bloodstream. Taking addictive drugs when pregnant means that your baby is highly likely to be born with a drug dependency. All street drugs should be avoided when you are pregnant. If you need help to give up, ask your caregiver for advice.

Alcohol in Pregnancy

There is no doubt that drinking heavily during pregnancy is not a good idea – it can cause brain and developmental damage to your baby. Alcohol can cross the placenta, so effectively your baby drinks when you do. Some women cannot bear the taste of alcohol while they are pregnant, which is probably nature's way of protecting the baby. As a result many women choose to abstain from drinking completely; however, the odd glass of wine is not considered harmful to the baby, so toasting the happy couple at a wedding shouldn't be a cause for concern.

Eating Properly

In pregnancy, women require an extra 300 calories above their normal daily intake to meet the needs of their growing baby. The quality of those calories is particularly important; your developing child requires an extra boost of a variety of vitamins and minerals. Most of these nutrients are best served up in your regular diet. Start making it a habit to check nutrition labels in the supermarket, and invest in a good pocket-sized nutrition guide to help you choose fresh or perishable produce and other items that are unlabelled.

You may find yourself eating more snacks in pregnancy, either to keep morning sickness at bay or because your growing baby is leaving less and less room for a full stomach. Smaller, more frequent mini-meals can also help combat indigestion and heartburn. Try protein-filled snacks such as peanut butter on wholewheat crackers or yogurt with wheatgerm.

Nutrition guidelines for pregnancy can seem like a dazzling array of do's and don'ts, and almost everyone you meet will have an opinion on each morsel you put near your mouth. Add to this the effects of nausea and cravings and it can seem like a minefield, but as long as you follow a few basic rules you should be fine. Remember, your caregivers can advise you if you have any queries, and you will be given some leaflets which explain things clearly.

· Eat a balanced diet – plenty of fresh fruit and vegetables – and cut down on processed foods, which are often packed with fat and sugar and not much else.

· Eat plenty of fibre – constipation is often a problem in pregnancy, but watch out for foods that make you bloated or flatulent.

· Eat about an extra 300 calories a day – forget about 'eating for two': a glass of milk and a snack should do it. Milk also provides much-needed calcium, so it's a great way to up your calorie intake. Light snacks can help keep nausea at bay, as well as providing extra calories.

· Take a folic-acid supplement throughout the first trimester – you shouldn't need other supplements unless your caregiver specifically advises you.

· Limit your caffeine intake – caffeine inhibits iron absorption, and can play havoc with your digestion. Cut down to one cup a day – although the very thought of tea or coffee makes many pregnant women queasy.

· Wash all fruit and vegetables.

· Avoid the following: unpasturized dairy produce, undercooked eggs, meat, poultry and patés, offal.

· Listen to your cravings – your body may be telling you what you need, but stick to the safety guidelines and don't overdo it!

 Many women drink herbal teas instead of caffeinated drinks, and these are usually considered safe. However, do not drink raspberry leaf tea, as this can trigger contractions.

Folic acid

Folica acid, or folate, is one of the B vitamins. A good intake of folic acid during the first trimester significantly reduces your baby's risk of developing a neural tube defect, such as spina bifida or anencephaly. A number of foods contain folic acid, and in addition, some foods, especially cereals, are fortified with folate. To be on the safe side, it is recommended that women take a supplement of folic acid when planning a baby if possible, and certainly during the first 12 weeks of pregnancy (when the baby's neural tube is forming).

Foods with folic acid include:

· dark green vegetables
· cereals, especially wholegrains. Some breads and cereals are fortified with folic acid – check the labels
· oranges, grapefruit, bananas
· beans and pulses

· milk and yoghurt
· yeast or malt extracts

Exercising Your Body

Women who work out regularly or participate in sports are often worried about whether or not they can continue their routine with a baby on board. In most cases, exercise is not only allowed, it's encouraged. However, the relaxing effects of progesterone during pregnancy make you more prone to injury, so go easy. All pregnant women, especially those in high-risk pregnancies and those who were inactive prior to pregnancy, should talk to their doctor about exercise options.

Vigorous team sports that pose a risk of injury to you or baby, such as netball or hockey, should be avoided. Scuba diving is also not advised because of the risk of decompression sickness. However, swimming, walking and cycling are ideal ways to stay fit throughout pregnancy. Your local gym or community health centre may also offer special exercise programmes geared toward the prenatal set.

Always stay well hydrated when you work out, and try to confine exercise to the coolest parts of the day in the summer months. An excessive rise in core body temperature (hyperthermia), particularly in the first trimester, has been associated with birth defects. If you feel yourself getting warmer than is comfortable, stop your exercise routine and cool down.

Using Medications

Sometimes women decide to self-treat colds and other illnesses with dietary supplements and herbal and botanical remedies in pregnancy, mistakenly assuming that medicine from a botanical source is inherently safe for their foetus. Remember: 'natural' doesn't necessarily mean harmless; herbs can be potent medicinal substances. Even seemingly benign substances like herbal tea have the potential to interact with other foods and medications and cause harm to your developing child. Always check with your doctor before taking anything medicinal, herbal or otherwise.

On Your Mind

Although physical wellness and mental health are often perceived as two separate and distinct things, the truth is that the mind and body are inextricably linked and what impacts one usually affects the other as well. This connection is particularly strong in pregnancy, as the rapid physical changes taking place alter the biochemical balance of the body and brain. Pregnancy is also a precursor to one of the biggest life-changing events there is – the arrival of a baby – and that alone is enough to stir up new and unexpected feelings.

Emotional Health

The hormonal changes that occur in pregnancy can have you feeling tearful one minute and irritable the next. And the emotions you experience, especially the negative ones, can be detrimental to your growing child. Depression, stress and anxiety may alter your eating and sleep patterns, robbing you and baby of the nutrients and rest you need. Clinical studies have found that depression and stress also have a direct impact on foetal growth and infant development. If you are feeling blue, you aren't alone; up to 10 per cent of women experience ongoing antepartum depression, and 70 per cent have had depressive symptoms at some point in their pregnancy. Yet women frequently feel guilty that they are feeling so bad during a period of their life that is supposed to be joyful, and for that reason many do not seek professional help.

If you're feeling hopeless, sad, tired, having trouble sleeping or losing interest in things that used to give you pleasure, you may be experiencing antepartum depression. Research has linked depression during pregnancy to preterm delivery, lower birth weight, developmental problems in infancy and a 50 per cent chance of developing postpartum depression after the baby is born. Don't wait – talk to your doctor about treatment options today.

Keeping Stress in Check

Pregnancy is a stressful time. A lot of it is positive, exciting stress as you plan for the baby. But you may also be feeling the pressures of impending financial and family responsibilities, fears of labour and delivery, and new career challenges. Trying to keep up with a hectic prepregnancy schedule as your body grows to a very large and unwieldy size is also a certain way to stress. In high enough amounts, the stress hormone cortisol can cross the placental barrier and have an impact on foetal brain development. It has also been linked to the development of high blood pressure in animal offspring studies. That's why it's essential to take time out for yourself throughout your pregnancy to decompress (see Chapter 4 for more on stress management).

Genetic Counselling

If you have a history of genetic disease or birth defects in your family, or are considered at risk for passing along a hereditary disorder based on your ethnic or racial background, your doctor or midwife may refer you to a genetic counsellor, another tool in the prenatal diagnostic arsenal. Genetic counselors certified by the American Board of Genetic Counseling have a CGC designation after their name, which indicates that they have passed a certification exam, have a graduate degree in genetic counseling, and have logged significant clinical training experience.

What It Is

A genetic counselor takes a detailed family and social history and creates a statistical analysis of your child's risk for acquiring genetic or birth defects. She will also provide you with information on the conditions in question and the risks and benefits of further testing, and will answer any questions you may have. Some of these tests may involve checking you or your partner for carrier genes, while others test the foetus (for more on diagnostic and screening tests see Chapter 5).

I'm 40 and pregnant with my second child. What are my chances of an uncomplicated pregnancy?
Women over age 35 have a higher risk for developing diabetes, high blood pressure and placental problems in pregnancy. There is also an increased risk of having a baby with a chromosomal disorder such as Downs syndrome – at age 40 your chances are 1 in 100. However, prenatal care can greatly reduce your risk of many birth defects and complications.

What It Isn't

Some women refuse genetic counselling on the grounds that they would never elect to terminate their pregnancy. However, genetic counselling isn't designed to be a 'survival of the fittest' venture, but rather a way to help you and your spouse or partner reach an informed decision. A genetic counsellor is trained to remain objective and not attempt to influence your choices. Many couples can and do continue a pregnancy, even after testing indicates their child will be born with a serious medical condition or birth defect. Advance knowledge allows a family to prepare emotionally, and to create a suitable environment for a special-needs newborn. It can also mean a better outcome for the child to have a medical support network already in place.

For more on genetic tests and screening, see Chapter 13.

Chronic Health Conditions

If you have a chronic health problem such as diabetes, asthma or heart disease, you will face some special challenges over the next nine months as your body adjusts to the major remodelling going on inside right now. Remember that your baby's health depends on your well-being, so staying on top of your treatment is essential. It's important to bring your primary health-care provider into the pregnancy picture as soon as possible (ideally, when you start planning your pregnancy).

Your doctor may adjust your medication or treatment regimen, and in most cases will want to follow your progress closely. You may also be referred to a perinatologist who specializes in high-risk pregnancies. See Chapter 13 for more on chronic illness and high-risk pregnancies.

Chapter 2

Month 1

During the first trimester of pregnancy, which lasts approximately 14 weeks from the first day of your last menstrual period, your body is hard at work forming one of the most intricate and complex works of nature. By the end of your first official month of pregnancy (six weeks after your last menstrual period, but four weeks since conception), your developing child will have grown an astonishing 10,000 times in size since fertilization.

Baby This Month

Making its longest journey until the big move nine months from now, your developing baby (called a zygote, or fertilized ovum) travels from the fallopian tube and into the uterus (or womb). After fertilization, the zygote begins a process of rapid cell division, and by day four it has formed a small solid cluster of cells known as a morula (after *moris,* Latin for 'mulberry'). The morula finishes the trip down the fallopian tube, reaching the uterus about three to four days after fertilization.

The Blastocyst

By day five or six your baby takes on its third name change in less than a week as the morula grows to a blastocyst. The blastocyst contains two distinct cell layers with a cavity at the centre. The inner layer will evolve into the embryo, and the outer layer will develop into the placental membranes – the amnion and the chorion. Within days, the blastocyst nestles into the nutrient-rich lining of your uterus (the endometrium) as implantation begins about a week after conception. Wispy fingers of tissue from the chorion layer, called chorionic villi, will anchor the blastocyst firmly to your uterine wall, where they will begin to build a network of blood vessels. These villi are the start of the placenta, a spongy oval-shaped structure that will 'feed' the foetus (via the umbilical cord) with maternal nutrients and oxygen throughout pregnancy.

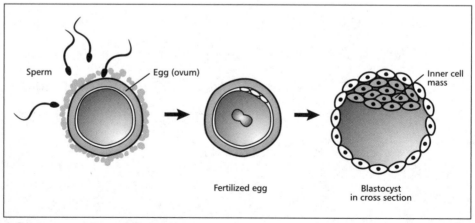

▲ From conception to blastocyst.

The Embryo

About 15 days after conception, the blastocyst officially becomes an embryo. Next to the embryo floats the yolk sac, a cluster of blood vessels that provide blood for the embryo at this early stage until the placenta takes over. The embryo is surrounded by a watertight sac called the amnion (or amniotic sac). The amniotic fluid that fills the sac provides a warm and weightless environment for your developing baby. It also serves as a sort of embryo airbag (or in this case, fluid bag), protecting baby from the bumps and bustle of your daily routine. Nature efficiently double-bags your baby, surrounding the embryo and the amnion with a second membrane called the chorion.

During this first four weeks of development, your embryo has laid the groundwork for most of its major organ systems. As the first month draws to a close, baby's heart is beating (although you won't be able to hear it for several weeks yet), lung buds have appeared, and construction of the gastrointestinal system and liver are well underway. The neural tube, the basis of the baby's central nervous system, has developed and the forebrain, midbrain and hindbrain are defined. He (or she) is starting to look more like a person, too. The first layer of skin has appeared, facial features are surfacing, and arm and leg buds – complete with the beginnings of both feet and hands – are visible. It's an amazing list of accomplishments, considering your baby is about the size of a raisin (less than 6mm/¼inch long).

Your Body This Month

From your tired and anxious mind to your busy bladder, all your body's systems may seem to be in overdrive during these early days of pregnancy. The first thing you will notice is the absence of your monthly menstrual period – in many cases, this is what tipped you off to your pregnancy in the first place. Your embryo is secreting the human chorionic gonadotropin (hCG) hormone into your system. In addition to interrupting menstruation, hCG signals the ovaries to produce the hormone progesterone until the eighth week of pregnancy, when the placenta takes over production.

▲ Now an embryo, your baby at month 1 of gestation.

Your Body Changes

At this point in your pregnancy, you might not notice any significant changes in shape and size. Although you aren't menstruating, you feel slightly bloated and your waistband may begin to feel a bit snug. Your breasts may also start to increase in size, and the areolas around your nipples may enlarge and darken. No period? Bigger breasts? This baby is doing wonders for you already! Now for the cloud around that silver lining – fuller breasts are often more tender in pregnancy (although a supportive sports bra can help).

You may also experience increased vaginal secretions similar to those you get premenstrually, another hormonal side effect. These typically last throughout pregnancy and may actually worsen in the third trimester, so stock up on panty liners now. Normal vaginal secretions in pregnancy are clear to white in colour, mucus-like and both odour- and pain-free. If you experience discharge that is thick, foul-smelling, off-colour or accompanied by itching, blood or pain, contact your doctor immediately, to rule out infection or other problems.

Some women experience minor vaginal blood flow, called spotting, as the embryo implants itself into the uterine wall. Because of the timing – seven to ten days after ovulation - it is often mistaken for the beginning of the menstrual period. The spotting, which usually lasts only for one or teo days, is pink to brown and may be accompanied by minor cramps.

What You Feel Like

Building a baby is hard work, and even though it's early in the process, it isn't unusual to feel tired and run down right now. If at all possible, try to grab a nap during the day. If that isn't feasible due to a full-time job or other young children at home, make an early bedtime a priority. Although it may run contrary to your nature to be sleeping away the daylight hours when you could be accomplishing one of the 75 other things on your to-do list, thinking of it as nap time for baby may help. Once you've started down the long road of sleepless nights that new motherhood brings, you'll be longing for the days of early bedtimes and frequent naps!

You may also find yourself spending more and more time in the toilet. You are urinating more frequently due to high levels of progesterone, which relax your bladder muscles. Unfortunately, frequent urination is one symptom that will likely remain with you throughout pregnancy as your baby grows and the uterus exerts more and more pressure on your bladder. Constipation may become a problem due to increased levels of progesterone; you also may experience problems if you're taking iron supplements (for more on easing constipation, see Chapter 6).

Your cardiovascular system is undergoing big changes now, as it adjusts to meet baby's growing demand for the oxygen and nutrients your blood is carrying. Circulating pregnancy hormones dilate, or expand your blood vessels to accommodate an eventual 50 per cent increase in blood volume. Your cardiac output, a measurement of how hard your heart is working to pump blood, increases by 30–50 per cent, while your blood pressure drops. This is why you may find yourself feeling faint. If you are dizzy or lightheaded, sit or lie down on your side as soon as possible. Try not to lie flat on your back, particularly later in pregnancy, as the pressure your uterus places on both the aorta and the inferior vena cava (two of the large blood vessels that help keep oxygen circulating to you and baby) will actually make the dizziness worse.

If episodes of fainting or dizziness persist, or are accompanied by abdominal pain or bleeding, contact your docter immediately. They could be symptoms of ectopic (or tubal) pregnancy, a potentially fatal condition where implantation occurs outside of the endometrial lining of the uterus (in the fallopian tubes). See Chapter 13 for more on ectopic pregnancy.

And then there's the most notorious of all pregnancy symptoms – morning sickness. Up to 80 per cent of women experience one or both of these symptoms at some point in their pregnancy. As you may know all too well by now, the more accurate term is morning, noon and night sickness; pregnancy sickness can happen at any time, and strikes with varying intensity. Many women find that their stomach starts to settle as the first trimester draws to a close (anywhere from week 12 to week 16), but for others the queasiness persists throughout the entire pregnancy. Pregnancy sickness and relief strategies are covered in depth later in this chapter.

At the Doctor

See your GP as soon as you know you are pregnant. He or she will confirm the pregnancy and make a booking appointment

If you haven't had a Pap smear in the last year, your provider may also take a vaginal swab of cells scraped from your cervix for this purpose. You may also be offered tests for STIs and HIV. For a detailed look at diagnostic and screening tests in pregnancy, go to Chapter 5.

Your doctor may supply you with educational brochures and pamphlets on prenatal care, nutrition, office policies and other important issues. There will be a lot of new information to absorb, so don't feel as though you have to study everything on the spot. However, do take everything home so you can read and refer to it later. Start a folder or notebook for keeping pregnancy information together, and store it near your bed or other favourite reading and relaxation spot for easy access. Add a pad of paper to your 'pregnancy portfolio' so you can jot down any questions for your doctor or midwife.

Remember, the dad-to-be is in on this pregnancy, too. By all means bring your spouse or partner to the doctor with you. In addition to providing moral support, he probably has just as many questions about baby as you do. He can also help you remember the things your provider tells you that seem to promptly leave your brain as soon as you leave the surgery.

Confirming Your Pregnancy

Modern home pregnancy tests are highly sensitive (many claim a 99 per cent or higher accuracy rate), and provide many women with a convenient and private way to confirm their pregnancy. However, juggling sticks, strips and tiny plastic cups while trying to decode the magic answer window does leave some room for operator error. If your doctor hasn't yet officially confirmed your pregnancy with a lab test, he or she will do so now at this first visit, typically with a urine test, although a blood (or serum) test may be used. The pregnancy test measures the amount of hCG in your system. Urine tests detect levels above 25–50 milli-international units per milliliter (mIU/mL), while the more sensitive serum tests can detect levels as low as 5–10 mIU/mL. Blood tests may be performed in cases where a urine test is negative but pregnancy is still suspected (usually in the early weeks). If the test is negative but you still think you may be pregnant, wait a few days, then take another test.

Because your urine will not start to contain hCG until after the embryo is implanted in the endometrial lining of the uterine wall, a home test will not always detect your pregnancy as early as it may claim.

Estimating Your Due Date

While pregnancy lasts approximately 280 days, or about nine calendar months, your estimated date of delivery (or EDD) is based on a ten 'lunar-month' pregnancy. Each month is four seven-day weeks. Why lunar months instead of following a good old-fashioned calendar? Lunar months are based on a 28-day menstrual cycle, which is considered the average cycle length.

It's important to remember that most providers determine gestational age (how far along you are) from the first day of your last menstrual period (called LMP). This means that you are officially two weeks pregnant at the moment of conception. How's that for an existential twist? Of course, if your cycle is longer or shorter than 28 days, or if you have an irregular menstrual period, some mathematic gymnastics are required. In addition, if you're hazy on the date of your LMP, the EDD could be harder to pinpoint. Refer to Appendix C for an estimated due date table.

Because this is all so confusing, your doctor probably makes good use of the preprinted EDD charts in her office. However, if you do have a regular 28-day cycle, you can work out your own EDD by taking the date of your last period, counting three months back, and then adding seven days. For example, if your last period began on 1 September, you would go back through August and July, and into June. Then add seven days to come up with an estimated due date of 8 June. An alternate method is to count 280 days (40 weeks) from the first day of your last period.

Learning the Ropes

At each appointment you provide a urine sample, are weighed and have your blood pressure taken. Other diagnostic and screening tests may also be administered throughout pregnancy (for more on these, see Chapter 5). Once you're in the examination room, you may or may not have to undress, depending on your doctor's policy and how pregnant you are. For your first prenatal visit you will probably don a gown for a full physical exam. Later, some doctors will simply ask you to move your clothing aside for a quick belly check and measure, while others prefer a more thorough examination (e.g. checking your heart rate, examining your feet for any swelling).

tips

Get to know the staff in your doctor's surgery. Not only will it make your visits a more pleasant experience, it provides you with an invaluable personal contact when you're trying to squeeze in an unexpected appointment or having trouble reaching your doctor.

When to Call the Doctor, Day or Night

At your first appointment, your doctor may discuss how patient phone calls are handled, both during the day and after hours.

Usually an answering service picks up after-hours calls and pages the doctor or midwife on duty, who then returns your call. In most group practices, doctors and nurses usually take turns covering nights and weekends, so you will get a call back from the on-call health team. If you aren't given any guidelines for reaching staff after hours, make sure you ask.

Call your doctor immediately if you experience any of the following list of symptoms:

- Abdominal pain and/or cramp
- Fluid or blood leaking from the vagina
- Abnormal vaginal discharge (e.g. foul-smelling, green or yellow)
- Painful urination
- Severe headache
- Impaired vision (e.g. spots or blurring)
- Fever over 38°C (100.4°F)
- Chills
- Excessive swelling of face and/or body
- Severe and unrelenting vomiting and/or diarrhoea

You should also become familiar with the signs of preterm labour (covered in Chapter 13). Some women hesitate to pick up the phone for fear that they're being oversensitive or a hypochondriac. While a good dose of common sense should be used in contacting your doctor after hours (for example, a call regarding the pros and cons of epidurals is probably not a good idea at 3 AM – unless you're in labour, of course), in most cases 'better safe than sorry' applies. Remember, you're heading this pregnancy team. Learn to trust your instincts. If something just doesn't feel right to you, make the call.

On Your Mind

Pregnancy, particularly a first pregnancy, is a time of great anticipation as you head out into uncharted waters. Now that you've been to your first prenatal appointment and have officially started this journey, you may be surprised to find yourself filled with conflicting emotions.

Elation and Excitement

If this is a planned pregnancy, particularly a long-fought-for and hard-earned one, you may be thrilled beyond belief. Of course, even the little surprises can be sources of great joy. You are creating a new and unique life of boundless potential. As a family, you will share your hopes, dreams, knowledge and love. This is one of the most important tasks – and special experiences – of your life. So excitement, and even a few cheers and whoops, is the order of the day.

If you haven't shared the good news with your other children or family members yet, look ahead to Chapter 11 for some tips.

Feeling drippy? Pregnancy hormones may have you producing excess saliva, a condition called ptyalism. Postnasal drip and/or congestion is another common side-effect of hormonal changes. Both of these may be at least partial contributors to an unsettled stomach or morning sickness.

Anxiety

Worries about the baby's health and the possibility of miscarriage are common fears early in pregnancy. If you've had a previous miscarriage, you may be walking on eggshells trying to second-guess every move you make. The good news is that knowing your history of miscarriage, your doctor will be following your progress closely.

Although it may be easier said than done, letting go of your anxieties, at least for a little while, is the best thing for you and your baby right now. Try designating a certain area of your home, like your bedroom, a 'worry-free' zone, and then stick to a vow to let your anxieties go when you are in that space. Use sounds, sights and smells to make it as comfortable and relaxing as possible. An aromatherapy candle you like, soft music or nature sounds and some soothing scenery in the form of photographs and posters can do wonders for your state of mind. (For more on miscarriage and problems in pregnancy, see Chapter 13.)

You may also be concerned about your ability to provide and care for your child. It's important to remember that good parents learn with experience, and by the experiences of others. The very fact that you're reading this book and getting regular prenatal care shows that you want the best for your baby. By the time your little bundle arrives, you'll be surprised at how much you've learned in the relatively short space of nine months.

Morning Sickness

Your stomach flutters, then lurches. As your mouth starts to water, you run for the bathroom for the fifth time today. Sound familiar? Morning sickness – called pregnancy sickness or nausea and vomiting of pregnancy

(NVP) by the medical profession – is arguably the most debilitating and prevalent of pregnancy symptoms. While most women find that NVP symptoms subside or stop as the first trimester ends, for some they continue into the second and even third trimester. If you're having twins or more, your NVP may also be longer and more intense.

The exact cause of NVP has not been pinpointed, but theories abound. Some possible culprits: the human chorionic gonadotropin (hCG) hormone that surges through your system and peaks in early pregnancy; a deficiency of vitamin B and B_6; hormonal changes that relax your gastrointestinal tract and slow digestion; and immune system changes. Another hypothesis is that morning sickness is actually a defense mechanism that protects both mother and child from toxins and potentially harmful micro-organisms in food. No matter what the cause is, it's a miserable time for all concerned.

I can't stand wearing what was my favourite perfume any more! Can pregnancy cause your nose to go haywire?
Pregnancy causes a heightened sensitivity to certain odours – coffee, cigarette smoke and fried foods are frequent offenders – that can contribute to stomach unrest. One theory is that these olfactory aversions are your body's way of keeping you away from substances that could harm your developing baby.

Remedies and Safety

The following treatments have been associated with some success in lessening symptoms of NVP in clinical trials. (Talk to your doctor or nurse before adding any new supplements to your diet.)

- Ginger. Ginger snaps and other foods and teas that contain ginger (*Zingiber officinale*) may be helpful in settling your stomach. Fresh ginger is best.
- Acupressure wristbands. Sometimes used to ward off motion and sea-sickness, these wristbands place pressure on what is called the P6, or Nei-Kuan, acupressure point. Available at most pharmacies, they are

an inexpensive and non-invasive way to treat NVP.
- Vitamin B and B₆. Thiamine (B₁) and B₆. Try eating snacks rich in B vitamins, such as bananas. It has been suggested that NVP is a sign of B vitamin deficiency.

Kava-aava (*Piper methysticum*), liquorice root (*Glycyrrhiza glabra*), rue (*Ruta graveolens*), Chinese cinnamon (*Cinnamomum aromaticum*) and safflower (*Carthamus tinctorius,* or saffron) are just a few of the many botanical remedies that are known to be dangerous in pregnancy. Don't take that supplement or cup of herbal tea without asking your doctor first.

Other treatments that women report as helpful include:

- **Eating smaller, more frequent meals.** An empty stomach produces acid that can make you feel worse. Low blood sugar causes nausea.
- **Choosing proteins and complex carbohydrates.** Protein-rich foods (e.g. yogurt, beans) and complex carbs (e.g. baked potato, whole grain breads) are good for the two of you and may calm your stomach.
- **Eat what you like.** Most pregnant women have at least one food aversion. If broccoli turns your stomach, don't force it. The better foods look and taste, the more likely they are to stay down.
- **Drink plenty of fluids.** Don't get dehydrated. If you're vomiting, you need to replace those lost fluids. Some women report better tolerance of beverages if they are taken between meals rather than with them. Turned off by water and juice right now? Try juicy fruits like watermelon and grapes instead.
- **Brush regularly.** Keeping your mouth fresh can cut down on the excess saliva that plagues some pregnant women. Breath mints may be helpful as well.

How to Cope

Constant queasiness and vomiting may have you wondering why on earth you got pregnant in the first place. Try to take solace in the fact that for most women, NVP is primarily a first-trimester affair. Stick close to home, and take it easy if at all possible. When staying home isn't an option, talk to your employer about allowing some flexibility with your work schedule. If your stomach is at its worst first thing in the morning, ask about starting later in the day on a temporary basis. Depending on your occupation, working from home on some days may be an option. For more on working through pregnancy, see Chapter 9.

Put together a morning-sickness survival kit for the car. Items to include: wet wipes, tissues, small bottle of water; travel-size toothbrush and toothpaste, a pack of gum or breath mints, water biscuits or crackers, and a bundle of large freezer bags. For longer trips, a mobile phone and a 'just-in-case' change of clothes are a necessity.

When It May Be More Than Morning Sickness

When your body can't get the energy it needs from food, it will start to metabolize stored fat. This condition, called ketosis, generates ketones that circulate in your bloodstream and can harm your foetus. Your doctor may test your urine for ketones if you're having severe and persistent nausea and vomiting.

0.3–3 per cent of pregnant women experience a severe form of morning sickness called hyperemesis gravidarum (excessive vomiting of pregnancy). If you can't keep any food or fluids down, are losing weight and are finding it impossible to function normally, you may be in this category. Although hospitalization is sometimes required for hyperemesis gravidarum, the treatment – intravenous fluids to restore fluid and electrolyte balance, and in some cases, antiemetics (to stop vomiting) – is relatively simple. If you are prescribed antiemetics, talk to your doctor about the safety data on the drug you are prescribed and any potential effects on the foetus.

Just for Dads

Fathers have their own unique role in pregnancy. While you may not be physically carrying this child (probably a source of enormous relief as you watch your partner struggle with morning sickness and other pregnancy fun), you are sharing the emotional weight of pregnancy, experiencing the same fears, joys and occasional bewilderment as your partner. You also have the added responsibility of being her primary source of support in many cases. In fact, this may be the first time in your lives when she is in charge of the manual labour and you're the emotional caregiver. Try to enjoy this new vantage point – think of it as training for life as a dad.

This Wild Ride Called Pregnancy

Although your partner might not look very pregnant yet, the chances are that she's acting that way. Mood swings, 'emotional lability' in medical terms, are the result of the many hormonal changes pregnancy brings, and may be one of the first things you notice. So if you're laughing together one minute and being yelled at the next, don't take it personally. It's all part of the package.

Morning sickness, particularly when it is severe, can be a disturbing part of pregnancy for men. Supporting your partner during this difficult time – making sure she gets adequate rest, taking care of household duties and catering to her food requests, no matter how odd they may seem – is the best way you can help both her and your child.

Fear of the Future

It's natural to feel nervous about providing for an utterly dependent and very tiny person. Practical matters, like being able to support a bigger family, may be dominating your thoughts right now. If you haven't done so already, talk to your spouse or partner about your concerns; the chances are that she shares many of the same anxieties as you do, and working together as a family is the best way to face them head-on.

Chapter 3

Family Matters

No matter what shape and size your current household is, a new baby in your home will touch your life in ways you never imagined. Just about every aspect of your daily routine is going to change – how you eat, sleep, play and work. As you wait to welcome your child to the world, use the time to lay the foundation for your new family circle.

Make Room for Baby

Kids are remarkably adaptable. They can thrive in just about any location, given a healthy and nurturing environment. They do need a safe space to grow in, however; babies in particular learn through exploring and experiencing their surroundings.

A Space of Their Own

Start thinking about where your baby will be sleeping (or not sleeping!) and playing so you can co-ordinate logistics and gear. Keep an open mind, however. Even if you can't wait to see your little angel peacefully dozing against his colour-co-ordinated crib sheets, you may have second thoughts about having him far away 'down the hall' once he arrives (especially when the 2 AM feeding rolls around).

Some parents choose to keep their newborn in their room, either in a crib or cot or in the parental bed – a somewhat controversial practice also called co-sleeping. Proponents of this say that it encourages breast-feeding, boosts milk production and provides a better bonding experience for parents and baby. Critics cite studies that conclude that bed sharing disrupts sleep patterns and increases the risk of sudden infant death syndrome (SIDS). However, factors such as sleep position, type of bedding and parental smoking and alcohol consumption raise the risk of cot death as well, and it isn't completely clear whether bed sharing in the absence of these risk factors still presents a significant hazard.

Make sure baby sleeps safe on a firm mattress, without soft bedding or duvets. Always place him on his back to sleep, and never share a bed with a baby after you have been drinking or if you are under the influence of drugs that alter consciousness.

Whatever you decide regarding sleeping arrangements (and you may not decide until you actually have her in your arms), if you have the space you're probably already laying plans for the baby's room. If you're torn about giving up your study for a nursery (after all, she's small – how much space can she need?), think about the baby basics (crib, changing area, dresser) plus all the inevitable *stuff* you're bound to acquire – stuffed animals, bouncy chairs, baby books – and the choice becomes clear.

If a nursery isn't an option due to the size of your home or financial considerations, there are several ways to give baby a place of her own. A folding screen (or two) or curtains hung from a ceiling track can be a creative way to close off part of a room. If you have the money but have limited room, think of building a wall for a more permanent partition.

Wherever it is, the baby's space should be well ventilated and insulated. Evaluate the area for safety hazards such as peeling paint, dangling blind cords and loose flooring. If there are doorstoppers installed, make sure they are one-piece; the rubber bumper on many models represents a choking hazard. When it comes time to purchase a cot, make sure that it has no decorative features that could potentially catch on clothing or trap the baby, and that the crib slats are a maximum of 60mm (2³/₈in) apart. The mattress should fit snugly against the sides.

Bye Bye MG, Hello People Carrier

Time to face the cold hard facts – that sporty two-seater just isn't going to be practical once you have both a baby and all her associated cargo to carry about town.

You don't need to run out and buy a 4WD, but you should cast a critical eye toward your current vehicle and make sure it meets both the practical and safety concerns of your growing family. Some things to look for:

· **Sit back and be safe.** The best place for any child is the back seat. If you have the choice, avoid SUVs or other vehicles that don't offer one.
· **Preferred seating.** Size matters, and so does shape. Make sure that your car seat fits properly in the vehicle and there is adequate room if you have more than one child to secure. Remember your little one will ride in a rear-facing car seat until he weighs 9kg (20lb) and is a year old.
· **Passenger air bag on/off switch.** If your new baby must ride in the front passenger seat and there is an air bag, there absolutely *must* be a switch that allows you to disengage the air bag on that side.

Air bags can save lives, but used improperly they can also cause serious injuries. A rear-facing infant seat places your child's head just inches from the air bag, which expands with tremendous force and speed – a potentially fatal combination. Make sure any air bags fitted can be switched off before fitting the baby's seat.

- **Skip the side air bag.** Side impact air bags can also pose a significant risk of head and neck injury to children. If the vehicle has an activated rear seat side air bag, make sure it has been adequately tested for safe use with children. Otherwise, have it deactivated.
- **Interior boot release.** If your car was manufactured after September 2001 it should have a release mechanism inside the boot to prevent curious children from becoming trapped inside. Retro-fitted release latches are available for cars without this feature.
- **Don't run hot and cold.** If your heating and cooling system is out of commission, now is the time to get it fixed. You may not mind sweating in summer, but an infant can quickly become overheated. The CDC recommends turning on the car air conditioner in weather 75°F or warmer, and firing up the heater when it dips below 50°F.
- **Accessorize.** Car seat belts and buckles left in the sun can also pose a hazard to infants, so consider a car seat cover or window and windshield sun screens, which are also useful in preventing your car interior from absorbing the sun's heat.

Other features that may be helpful but aren't absolutely essential include built-in child car seats and safety door locks.

In hot weather, a car without air conditioning can reach extremely high temperatures in a matter of just a few minutes, even with the windows open a crack. Because of his small size, a baby's core body temperature rises quickly on a warm day – up to five times faster than that of an adult – and potentially fatal heat-related illness is a serious risk.

Babyproofing

Now that you have car safety covered, take a look at potential hazards inside your home.

Although your home safety efforts will undoubtedly pick up steam as your child gets mobile and starts exploring her surroundings, there are some basic things you can do now to protect her in infancy and beyond.

- **Register for recalls.** Take the time to fill out those registration and guarantee cards for all the baby gear you've received. If a safety recall of the product occurs, the manufacturer will be able to notify you.
- **Ban cigarettes.** You already know how dangerous it is to smoke during pregnancy, but did you know that secondhand smoke, particularly in a closed home environment, is harmful to your baby's health? Tobacco is also toxic when eaten; since babies put just about everything in their mouths, that's just one more good reason to make your home a tobacco-free zone.
- **Get the lead out.** Lead paint is a major hazard to small children. When ingested, either by eating paint chips or breathing lead dust, it can cause CNS damage and a host of other health and developmental problems. Lead solder used in some older plumbing systems can also pose a risk. If you haven't done so already, contact a lead inspector certified by the state and/or the Environmental Protection Agency (EPA) to test your home for the presence of lead and to advise you on abatement procedures, if necessary.
- **Rearrange the furniture.** Block off electrical cables and buy plastic protectors to seal up open sockets. Put pads on sharp table corners to protect baby from injury. Evaluate your home from a baby's eye view (about 1m/3ft off the floor for good measure), and move anything dangerous, expensive or breakable to higher ground.
- **Practise.** Some old habits – like leaving the toilet seat up – are hard to break. It will be easy to be vigilant later if you get accustomed to baby-safe behaviour now. A few new routines to try out: store medications, cleaning products and other toxic substances out of a child's reach; store plastic bags in a latched cabinet; and make sure all members of the household leave the toilet seat (and lid) down.

Rights and Entitlements

Having a baby is an expensive business – not many parents would argue with that. As well as the basic 'start-up' costs of the equipment you will need (not to mention a lifetime of clothes, toys, music tuition for your budding Mozart, designer trainers, driving lessons and university fees), you are probably going to experience a significant drop in household income. This can come as a shock to even the best prepared parents-to-be, so it's vital to know what you are entitled to.

Maternity rights in Britain are now the best they have ever been. In addition, many employers offer packages that are far better than the legal requirement, so do ask what is available.

Get Prepared

Tell your employer as soon as you know you are pregnant. If you delay notifying your employer of your intentions, you may lose some of your entitlements, and as your pregnancy progresses you will have other things to think about. You may not want anyone to know you are pregnant early on 'just in case', but you can tell the personnel department in confidence and make it clear that your pregnancy is not general knowledge. Some women worry that announcing they are pregnant will prejudice their career, but remember that it is illegal for your employer to discriminate against you because of your pregnancy.

Your Basic Rights

· All employees are entitled to paid time off for antenatal appointments, including antenatal classes.
· You cannot be treated unfairly, dismissed or made redundant because you are pregnant.
· You should be allowed to take sick leave without affecting your maternity entitlement.
· Free prescriptions and dental care throughout pregnancy and for one year afterwards.
· You are entitled to child benefit for your baby once he or she is born.

If you have any problems regarding your rights and entitlements, ask your caregivers for advice.

Maternity Leave

All working women are entitled to 26 week's maternity, regardless of length of employment or hours worked. Statutory maternity pay for this time is paid at 90 per cent of your average earnings for six weeks, then you receive £100 per week for the remaining 20 weeks.

If you have worked for your employer for at least 26 weeks prior to the 15th week before you are due, you are entitled to a further 26 weeks' unpaid leave – meaning that you can take 52 weeks off if you choose (and can afford) to do so.

If you are self-employed you can apply for Maternity Allowance, which is paid by the government.

You must give your employer at least four weeks' notice of your intention to take maternity leave, but it is courteous to give as much notice as possible.

You may want to work until very late in your pregnancy, but there are no guarantees of how you will feel, especially if you have to commute a long distance. Keep your plans flexible.

Paternity Leave

New fathers are entitled to two weeks' leave after the birth of each child. This is normally paid at £100 per week.

Unpaid Parental Leave

This is available to all mothers and fathers (including adoptive parents) who have been working for the same employer for a year. For each child, a parent is allowed a total of 13 weeks' unpaid leave up until the child's fifth birthday in addition to paid annual leave. If your child has a disability, you may be entitled to further leave – ask your doctor or health visitor if this affects you.

Financial Planning for a Bigger Family

Cost Comparisons

Clueless about baby care costs? Do a little detective work and make a reconnaissance mission to the supermarket to gather prices on nappies, baby wipes and other essentials. If you're considering day care or an in-home childminder, now is a good time to get information and monthly cost estimates. As usual, other parents are an excellent source of tips and leads to the best resources in your area.

In a week, the average baby goes through about 60–80 nappy changes. That's a potential pileup of 4,160 nappies in the first year alone! If you're using disposable ones, get prices for cases of nappies at the local discount store, since bulk purchases are typically cheaper.

Setting Savings Goals

So now that you've worked out what you'll be spending, what practical use do you put it to? Lay out your current spending habits, including basic monthly bills like utilities and housing, debts that can be downsized (e.g. credit cards and car payments), transport costs, food and household goods, health care and discretionary/disposable income.

Accounting for everything in black and white will give you a much clearer picture of where you're spending goes and the size of any gap between income and expenses. It can also help you work out big-picture questions like whether you have the financial means to switch to a part-time schedule at work.

When the time comes to balance your home budget, be realistic in your planning and prudent when you eliminate discretionary purchases; taking sandwiches to work each and every day for the next three years is a noble goal, but a weekly or biweekly meal out with colleagues could pay off in other ways. Give yourself a little breathing room for unforeseen emergency expenses, such as a malfunctioning household appliance or car repairs. A little scrimping here, one less latté a week there, and you'll find budgeting easier than you thought.

Lifestyle Changes, or Stating the Obvious

Your baby's arrival will transform just about everything you think, say and do. This sea change is probably most evident in first-time parents, who up until now have been enjoying the child-free pursuits of quiet dinners, X-rated films and even the occasional wild night out with the girls or boys. Even those mums and dads who are expecting a second or subsequent child will have big adjustments ahead, with new challenges like siblinghood and advanced parental multitasking (e.g. encouraging one child to use his napkin while preventing the other from eating hers). Don't look at it as an end, but rather a new and infinitely more rewarding chapter in your life. You may even find some family pastimes you had never considered before.

Sharing Pregnancy with the Dad-to-Be

With the big focus on mum and her growing belly, it's easy for dads to get overlooked in the pregnancy drama. Remind your significant other that you're in this together. If he isn't quite sure of his role in this new adventure yet, he could be looking to you for cues. Encourage him to join you at prenatal checkups, as well as to share pregnancy education and experiences like the first kicks. You should also try to pencil in some special couple time to 'talk' to baby, contemplate names and share your hopes and dreams about your family's future.

From Two to Three

The new person in your life has already started competing for your attention, changing your eating and sleeping patterns and perhaps slowing down your pace. Unexpected emotions may surface between you and your partner as your pregnancy progresses. He may feel pangs of jealousy at the loss of your being a couple and your focus on the baby. On the flip side, you may be feeling as if you're playing second fiddle to your foetus as he questions the safety of every move you make. Such growing pains are normal. Try to talk about your feelings, and approach parenting (even now) as a team effort.

Some dads are intimidated by the size and vulnerability of an infant, and as a result pass most of the child-care responsibilities on to the mother, a potential lose-lose situation for both of you. If he is feeling uneasy about his lack of previous experience in the child-care arena, suggest a few tag-team babysitting sessions for a niece or nephew or a friend's child to build his confidence.

The Bond of Parenthood

Pregnancy can bring a couple closer together than they ever imagined, but it can also present new frictions in your relationship. The aches and pains of pregnancy would push even the most even-tempered woman to her limits. Add to that a healthy surge of oestrogen and progesterone, and you have the recipe for major mood swings. Other stressors, like a tepid sex life and financial fears, can also stir the pot. Try to approach these temporary changes with understanding and empathy for your partner, and a healthy sense of humour if at all possible.

Strange but true – men can have pregnancy symptoms too. Known as couvade, this sympathy pain phenomenon may have your significant other experiencing nausea, fatigue, weight gain and mood swings. What's behind it? Anxiety associated with impending fatherhood is suspected by some, but a Canadian study found that men experiencing couvade had distinct hormonal changes that mirrored their pregnant partners.

Single Mums and Support

If you're a single mother-to-be by choice or by circumstance, you aren't alone. Pregnancy and birth are physically and emotionally challenging experiences. As a single mum, you may also have the added baggage of financial, career and custody concerns weighing on you. Dealing with the stress positively is important to you and your baby's health.

Don't fly solo if you don't have to. Enlist a family member or close friend to accompany you on prenatal visits, childbirth classes and the birth itself. A birthing partner can also be a wonderful source of support for labour and delivery. If at all possible, make arrangements for a live-in companion for the first few postpartum weeks as well.

An Eye to the Future

It may seem worlds away now, but things like school, parks and playgroups are waiting just around the corner. Don't rush the early years, but as you talk to other parents and families in your neighbourhood, start to gather information on the resources available in your area. If you are moving to a bigger home in anticipation of your new arrival, be sure to investigate the school district performance and community resources as part of your house-hunting now to save yourself another move in five years.

Kids in Community

The community you raise your child in will play a large part in shaping her values, beliefs and personality. Of course, you will be the gatekeeper for his early exposures to the outside world, but schools, playgroups and community services that reinforce your value system will make parenting your older child a group effort rather than a dictatorship. Just as important is your personal investment of time and talents you return to these same institutions.

It's almost never too early to get involved with a playgroup. Your baby will probably enjoy playing with you and observing other kids in a group setting from just a few months old. Investigate what's already available in your area, or talk to some parents and mums-to-be in your area about starting up something new once baby arrives. Laying the foundation for friendships and positive community relationships now will help your child flourish.

Faith and Family

New parents often find themselves exploring their roots and reconnecting with their own childhood. Even if your family is far away, you can still share the special moments of your pregnancy and birth through photos, videotapes and phone calls. Sharing the parenting experience across generations can be a powerful experience that forges a special new bond between mother, child and – ultimately – grandchild.

When it was just the two of you, spirituality may have taken a back seat in your busy lives. Now that you are going to have a child to raise and educate, the traditions and values of your faith, whatever it may be, are going to take on a new dimension. If you and your partner come from different religious backgrounds, this question holds special significance. Will you choose one organized religion over the other, or expose your child to both faiths? If you're concerned about christening or baptism, an inter-faith baptismal service that respects the traditions and beliefs of two-religion families may be an option. The important thing is to open up communications and talk about your expectations now.

Chapter 4

Month 2

You've made it into the second month, or weeks six to ten, of your pregnancy. By the end of this month, your baby will have out-grown its embryonic development and matured into a foetus. Your body is changing rapidly – you may start to feel pregnant now, if you didn't before.

Baby This Month

Your unborn child has now advanced from raisin to raspberry size – about 12mm (^{1}/2in) in length. By the end of the month, he or she will be about 25mm (1in) long (a large grape). The foetus is lengthening and straightening out of the shrimp-like, curled form it held last month. The tail she was sporting disappears around week eight and her closed eyes start to move from the sides of the head to their permanent location. The face is further defined by a nose and jaw, and the buds of 20 tiny baby teeth are present in the gums by week ten. The palate and vocal cords also form around this time.

*f*act

Boy or girl? Girl or boy? Your child will keep you guessing for at least a few more weeks. While external sex organs begin to differentiate this month, they won't become visible on ultrasound until around week 16-20 (and then only with some foetal co-operation). If you're scheduled for an amniocentesis, the gender of your child can be determined at that time. Then again, you may enjoy the element of surprise!

Important organ systems are nearly completed by the end of month 2. The right and left hemispheres of your baby's brain are fully formed, and brain cell mass grows rapidly. Soft bones begin to develop, and the liver starts to manufacture red blood cells until the bone marrow can take over the job in the third trimester.

Your unborn baby is also giving his brand-new organs a workout: heart chambers form, the pancreas begins to produce insulin, and the liver secretes bile. The stomach produces gastric juices, while the intestines, which have developed in the umbilical cord, move up into the abdomen by the end of the month.

Floating in about 10 teaspoons of amniotic fluid, your baby has plenty of room to flex the muscles she is now developing. Because of her small size and spacious accommodations, the chances are that you won't notice these movements now. At about 18–20 weeks, when the second trimester is in full swing and her quarters become a bit closer, you will feel the first flutterings, known as quickening.

If you are at risk of passing on a chromosomal abnormality or hereditary health condition to your child, you may choose to be scheduled for a chorionic villus sampling (CVS) at the end of this month. A CVS is typically administered between weeks 10 and 12, and involves taking a small sample of placental tissue for laboratory analysis. See Chapter 5 for details on CVS procedures and genetic testing.

▲ At the end of this month, your baby is officially a foetus.

Your Body This Month

If you weren't feeling very pregnant last month, you are probably starting to now. About midway through this month, hCG levels will begin to peak and then slowly decline as the placenta starts to produce the pregnancy hormones progesterone and estradiol. The ebb and tide of your hormones will trigger a few new pregnancy symptoms this month.

Your Body Changes

Even though you may not have put on any additional weight yet, your growing uterus is pushing the boundaries of your waistline. On average, most women gain 1.2–2.5kg (2.5–5lb) in the first trimester.

Changes in skin and hair are common in pregnancy. Hair that was fine and thin may become thick and shiny during pregnancy, and that fabled pregnancy 'glow' may actually be your flawless, blemish-free complexion. On the other end of the spectrum, acne problems and hair breakage and thinning may occur.

Chloasma, also known as melasma, may cause a mask-like darkening or lightening of your facial skin. Freckles and moles are prone to darkening, as well as other pigmented areas of your skin (e.g. areolas). To minimize chloasma and other hyperpigmentation, use a good sunscreen (factor 30 or higher) to cover exposed skin when you're out in the sun.

Will colouring my hair hurt my baby?
To date, there is no conclusive evidence that hair colour use in pregnancy is dangerous. If you are concerned over a possible risk, you can choose a vegetable-based or temporary colour treatment until baby is born. Some experts also recommend not using any chemical hair treatments during the first trimester.

Your gums may start to bleed when you brush your teeth, a condition known as pregnancy gingivitis. Make sure you floss and brush regularly, to keep your teeth and gums healthy. A warm salt-water rinse may soothe swollen gum tissues (ask your doctor first if you have a history of high blood pressure). Now is a good time to book a thorough cleaning with your dentist; in a few months, leaning back in a dental chair will be uncomfortable, if not impossible.

What You Feel Like

The stomach rumblings of the first month continue, and an increase in nausea and vomiting may actually occur as hCG levels peak toward the end of this month. On the plus side, your NVP may start to get better in the coming weeks as hCG levels wane. If you're one of those lucky women who do not experience morning sickness at all, you're probably not escaping the feelings of fatigue. Take the hint your body is giving you, and take time out to rest.

Other symptoms that may start or continue this month include:

- Frequent urination
- Tender, larger breasts
- Increased vaginal discharge
- Occasional dizziness or faintness
- Indigestion or wind
- Headaches
- Nasal congestion and/or runny nose
- Increased saliva

If you have a cat, hand over litter duties to someone else. Toxoplasmosis, a parasitical infection passed on by infected cat faeces and by undercooked meat, has the potential to cause brain damage and other medical problems in your unborn child. Cats also frequent gardens and sandpits, so wear gloves, and wash your hands thoroughly after working outside.

Get the Most Out of Doctor's Appointments

If you are scheduled for a check-up, bring along that list of questions that have come up since your last visit. Again, write these down when they come to you and your partner, so you won't have to rely on your memory in the surgery. And make sure your questions are answered before you leave; although it's nice to be asked if you have any concerns, in the busy atmosphere of a large practice your doctor may occasionally forget. Stop her before she finishes the appointment, and let her know you have a few questions. Never feel that you're being pushy or overbearing (remember, you're leading this team). In most cases, she will do what she can to educate you and reduce any anxieties. If she doesn't, it's never too late to find someone who will.

On Your Mind

Now that you're feeling more symptoms of pregnancy, the reality of impending parenthood may suddenly hit home. 'So much to do, so little time', you may be thinking. Understanding and recognizing your emotional changes can help you better control your stress levels.

Mood Swings

Find yourself laughing hysterically or sobbing uncontrollably? If you're normally the balanced type, these emotional outbursts can be downright alarming. You aren't losing control or losing your mind, you're experiencing the normal mood swings of pregnancy. Although this emotional lability may continue throughout pregnancy, it is typically strongest in the first trimester as you adjust to many changes.

Given the transformation your body is going through and the accompanying aches and pains, you have every right to be difficult. In fact, when you combine your physical discomforts with the spectrum of emotions you're experiencing as motherhood approaches, you've got a licensce to be hell on wheels. Of course, no one is happy when that happens (just ask your partner), so take steps now to reduce your stress level and achieve some balance.

Stress and Stress Management

It's easy to get stressed over what may seem like an overwhelming amount of preparation. Your body is already working overtime on the development of your child; try to keep your commitments and activities at a reasonable level to prevent mental and physical overload.

Controlling outside stress is even more important when your pregnant body is under the physical stress of providing for an unborn baby. And added psychological stress can make the discomforts of pregnancy last longer and feel more severe.

Some traditional stress control methods, such as relaxation techniques involving certain strenuous yoga positions or martial arts, for example, are not appropriate for pregnant women. You should also not try fad diets, herbal preparations or over-the-counter medications (which are generally not good stress control methods in any case). When in doubt, check with your doctor or midwife.

Anxiety may also have an impact on your child's health. An increase of corticotropin-releasing hormone (CRH), a stress-related substance produced by the brain and the placenta, has been linked to preterm labour and low birth weight. Research has also suggested a possible connection between first-trimester maternal stress and congenital malformations.

As you rush to get everything 'just so', remember that your little one is not going to care if the cot matches the dresser, but he will feel the effects of your excess tension. Keeping it all in perspective is important. So is taking steps to decompress when you do feel the pressure building.

Effective stress management involves finding the right technique for *you*. Relaxation and meditation techniques (e.g. progressive muscle relaxation, yoga with your doctor's consent), adjustments to your work or social schedule, or carving out an hour of 'me' time each evening to decompress are all ways you can lighten your load. Exercise is also a great stress-control method, but make sure you get your doctor's approval regarding the level of exercise that is appropriate for you.

Dressing for Two

Finding maternity clothes that are fashionable, that fit, that grow comfortably with you and that don't cost a fortune can be a challenge.

Start out by deciding how much you want to spend; if you blow your whole clothing budget on a few items, you're going to be awfully limited in your choice.

A few other things to keep in mind while you develop your wardrobe:

- **Consider your laundry threshold.** Check the labels and make sure that the care instructions mesh with your lifestyle. Hand-washing your delicates may not top your priority list right now. And make sure you get enough maternity pieces so you aren't washing the same three outfits constantly.
- **Mix and match.** Try to build on what you already own by adding pieces that will work well in a variety of combinations.
- **Keep your sense of style.** Although maternity clothes are getting more fashionable in response to women's needs, there are still plenty of overalls festooned with ruffles and appliqués, 'I'm With Foetus' slogan T-shirts and similar maternity monstrosities out there. Buy what you like; even if it takes a little searching, it will be worth it.
- **Built to last?** You'll only be wearing these clothes for a matter of months, so they don't need to be made to withstand a natural disaster. However, if you're planning on stretching their shelf life through another pregnancy, spending a little more on well-made, durable attire is more economical in the long run.

Look Good... Feel Good

Dressing well can improve your mood and self-image at a time when they may be shaky. Notice it's dressing *well*, not necessarily dressing up, in whatever your unique style sense calls for. That may mean a favourite jogging suit for running errands or a little (or big) black dress for a night out. Don't forget to purchase some nice clothes or pyjamas for your take-it-easy days. Even when you're throwing up and miserable, slipping on something cozy can comfort your soul, if not your stomach.

Shopping by Due Date

Think about the time of year when you'll be delivering, especially if you live in a region with an inconsistent climate. Being nine months' pregnant in the dog days of summer wearing the woollen trousers you bought in midwinter will not be a good thing. To bridge the seasonal shifts, buy clothing that can be layered – peeled down for summer and piled on for winter. Invest in mix-and-match pieces in breathable fabrics that are adaptable to temperature changes.

Beg, Borrow and Hire

What could you possibly find in your partner's closet? Plenty, if you use a little imagination. Oversized work shirts and a Hawaiian shirt or two if you're feeling adventurous. Even some of his chinos or other casual trousers may be a good fit in the early months of pregnancy, when you're too big for your old trousers, yet not quite to maternity clothes stage. If you're just starting to show in late summer, but want to save your clothing budget for autumn and winter weather attire, borrow a pair or two of his cargo shorts to fill the gap.

If you and your partner aren't a good match for size, ask formerly pregnant friends and family for contributions. Take what you're offered – graciously. Even if it doesn't look quite 'you' at the outset, try matching it with some of your own pieces and accessorizing; the diversity may do your meagre wardrobe some good.

There is also a new breed of maternity clothing boutique, where for a monthly or weekly fee you can hire a selection of outfits to get you through pregnancy. The biggest benefit – more variety in your wardrobe, since you can switch clothing on a regular basis. The downside – if you're planning on a subsequent pregnancy, you won't have anything to keep and use again for your investment.

Dressed for Success

Women who work in an office or other professional environment have the added challenge and expense of finding clothes for work and play. Because of their limited lifespan in most women's closets, maternity clothes make great secondhand or charity shop fodder. You may be surprised at some of the bargains you uncover. Consignment stores that deal specifically in maternity wear are also becoming more commonplace; check your Yellow Pages to see if there is one near you.

Just for Dads

Things get interesting this month as you both get familiar with the weird but wonderful world of the pregnant body. Step right up and witness the amazing expanding belly! Thrill to the fantastic swelling bustline! Dare to brave the snores and thrashes of the mother-to-be, as she tries to find comfort in her natural sleeping habitat! This truly is the greatest show on earth.

Her Changing Body

Getting your libidos in synch during pregnancy can be a challenge. If she's experiencing nausea and vomiting right now, the chances are she's not feeling too sexy. On the other hand, for some women the hormonal onslaught of pregnancy has their sexuality in overdrive. You too may feel a similar range of emotions as the pregnancy progresses. Although you may never have thought it possible, fears of somehow hurting the baby during intercourse and a new perception of your partner as a mother may have you shying away from the bedroom. Or, you may find her physical metamorphosis and composure and strength, despite it all, a highly sensual experience.

So what do you do if you aren't on the same sexual wavelength? First of all, be sympathetic to the physical demands on her body right now, and remember this is a temporary situation. She may be feeling insecure about her appearance, or just awkward and clumsy as her body grows. Stress and anxiety can also douse her sex drive. Reassure her that she's still beautiful, perhaps even more so, and try to lighten her load by helping out more around the house and taking over some of the tasks that may be getting difficult for her.

Unless your doctor has told you otherwise it is perfectly safe to continue having sex throughout your pregnancy, although the effect of pregnancy on libido varies wildly from day to day, from woman to woman (and from man to man). However, if you have a history of miscarriage or bleeding in pregnancy, or if you have placenta praevia you should abstain from sex. Once your waters have broken avoid penetrative sex.

If she's looking for love but you aren't, look at the reasons behind your feelings. Is safety a concern? Sex is safe and normal if the pregnancy is progressing normally. The baby is well protected in the uterus.

If you're thinking 'mummy' every time you see your partner and her baby bulge, you may have a harder time getting past your aversion to sexual intimacy. The most important thing is for you both to talk about it and discuss your feelings openly and honestly. Ignoring the problem will breed frustration and anger.

If you do agree to put sex on the back burner for a while, it doesn't mean a moratorium on romance. Bring her flowers, treat her to a weekend break, or just cook a special dinner one night and spend the evening talking about the future. Above all, enjoy each other and keep your relationship healthy.

Sympathy Pains

Every day she seems to have a new and interesting pregnancy symptom to report. Suddenly, you're feeling them too. Sympathetic pregnancy symptoms, known as couvade, are actually a fairly common occurrence. It's estimated that up to 65 per cent of men experience at least one or more pregnancy symptoms during their partner's pregnancy, including nausea, backache, weight gain and difficulty sleeping. The cause is likely multifaceted – a combination of psychological, social and possibly even biological factors. They do say that misery loves company; take it as a signal to have some rest and recuperation time together.

Chapter 5

Diagnostic Tests and Screening

You'll be poked, prodded, swabbed, scraped and scanned throughout your pregnancy. All these tests have a purpose, of course – a healthy mum and baby. This chapter gives you a rundown of what you have to look forward to, and what it all means.

Routine Checks

Antenatal care varies according to your circumstances and where you live, but generally routine tests involve weight, the size of the baby and your uterus, and a urine check. You will also be asked about any pregnancy symptoms or discomforts you are experiencing. You may also be offered internal examinations, especially towards the end of pregnancy to check that the cervix is ripening in preparation for birth. Your belly will be examined. Just how depends on where you are in your pregnancy, but you might expect a regular measurement of your fundal height (the top of your uterus) starting sometime in the second trimester, and an external check of the baby's position in the third trimester.

Urine Tests

You'll give a urine sample at each prenatal visit for urinalysis. Your surgery or lab will test your urine for ketones, protein and glucose at each visit, and may also check for the presence of any bacteria.

Depending on the protocol followed in your doctor's surgery, you may be asked to bring a fresh urine specimen to your appointment, or provide one upon your arrival. In either case, it's a good excuse to get some of those extra fluids your body and baby need right now. Down a bottle of drinking water on the way to your checkup so you can easily provide a sample, but don't overdo it or you may not make it without a pit stop.

Ketones

Ketone bodies are substances produced when the body is getting insufficient fuel from food intake and has to metabolize fat for energy. The result is a process known as ketosis, and the resulting ketones spill into the urine. Ketones may appear in pregnancy if you're suffering from severe nausea and vomiting, and they are a sign that you may require intravenous nutrition. They can also be a byproduct of gestational diabetes when blood sugars get too high, and can lead to a potential life-threatening complication called diabetic ketoacidosis (DKA).

Protein

Excessive protein (albumen) in the urine can be a sign of pre-eclampsia (also known as toxaemia or pregnancy-induced hypertension). It is also a possible indication of urinary tract infection (UTI) or renal (kidney) impairment. The presence of white blood cells in urine can be an indication of infection as well.

The kidneys are responsible for filtering waste products and fluids from the bloodstream into urine. Their function is also closely tied to blood-pressure regulation. As the volume of fluid in the bloodstream goes up with a blood-pressure increase (hypertension), the kidneys must work double time to clean and filter the blood. Eventually, the skyrocketing blood pressure threatens to damage the nephrons (filtering units of the kidneys) and the kidneys in turn cause the blood pressure to rise even further because they aren't able to adequately clear fluids. Be familiar with the warning signs of pre-eclampsia, which are covered in Chapter 13.

Glucose

Glucose, or sugar, in the urine (called glycosuria) may be a sign of gestational diabetes mellitus (GDM). It's normal to spill a small amount of sugar into the urine in pregnancy, but consistent high levels along with other risk factors raise a red flag that GDM may be present.

Urine Culture

Your urine will be analyzed and cultured for the presence of bacteria at your first prenatal visit, and again during pregnancy if symptoms of a urinary tract infection (e.g. burning during urination, strong-smelling urine) appear.

Other Blood Tests

Your blood type and rhesus, or Rh, factor will be determined at your first prenatal visit. An Rh factor is either positive or negative. If your Rh is positive, no treatment is necessary. If you are Rh negative, you are at risk for Rh incompatibility with the blood type of your baby. Rh incompatibility occurs when your unborn baby is Rh positive and your Rh negative blood combines with hers. When this happens, your immune system may try to fight off the baby as an intruder, causing serious complications. Receiving rhogain will prevent this from happening.

Blood tests also determine whether or not you are immune to German measles (rubella). German measles can cause birth defects, especially if you contract the infection during the first trimester, and can cause cataracts, heart defects and deafness in offspring. A majority of women have been exposed to the rubella virus or have been vaccinated against it before becoming pregnant, however, and immunity lasts a lifetime.

An HIV, hepatitis B, or syphilis test may also be done on your blood. For more on the testing of sexually transmitted diseases (STDs), see 'Swabs and Smears: Sexually Transmitted Diseases' below.

Blood tests can also screen for inherited anaemia in at-risk populations. For example, couples of African, Caribbean, Eastern Mediterranean, Middle Eastern and Asian descent are at risk for sickle cell anaemia. Families of Greek, Italian, Turkish, African, West Indian, Arabian or Asian descent may be screened for the thalassemia trait; if both father and mother are carriers, there is a chance that the foetus could develop the blood disease thalassemia major.

Swabs and Smears

More bodily fluid tests will be taken throughout pregnancy, particularly at the initial booking appointment. You may be offeredone or more of the following examinations. Remember: tests are offered to give you and your caregivers a clearer view of your pregnancy. Do not feel forced into having a test if you do not want it.

Pap Smear

Unless you've had one within the last year, your doctor may give you a Pap smear at your initial prenatal visit. During your pelvic exam, she will scrape a small sample of cells from your cervix using a spatula-like instrument. The cells are sent to a lab for microscopic analysis.

An abnormal Pap smear tells your doctor that something is going on with your cervix that requires further examination. While cervical cancer and pre-cancerous spots are a possibility, it is also quite possible that a simple vaginal infection or inflammation of the cervix is behind an abnormal Pap smear. STDs, particularly the human papillomavirus (HPV), can also cause irregularities. A closer look with another pelvic exam should tell your doctor, and you, more.

Group B Strep

Group B streptococcus (GBS) is a bacterium that can cause serious infections in a newborn baby – including pneumonia and meningitis. If a pregnant woman tests positive for it, she is usually prescribed intravenous antibiotics during labour and delivery to prevent transmission to her baby.

Swabs of both the rectum and vagina are taken and cultured (put in a medium that will allow the bacteria to grow if it is present).

Sexually Transmitted Diseases (STDs)

It is recommended that all pregnant women be screened for sexually transmitted diseases – chlamydia, gonorrhea, hepatitis B, HIV and syphilis – because of their potentially devastating effects on a foetus. HIV, hepatitis B and syphilis testing require a blood draw, while chlamydia and gonorrhea are tested with a polymerase chain reaction (PCR) test. You may be offered some of these tests, based on your medical history and perceived risk factors. If you'd like to be tested for all, ask your doctor.

Chlamydia, gonorrhea and syphilis are caused by bacteria and can be treated with antibiotics. Viral infections such as hepatitis B and HIV cannot be cured in the mother, but precautionary measures can greatly decrease the risks of passing on the disease to her child during labour and delivery.

Ultrasounds

The test that most women look forward to – the ultrasound – gives you your first glimpse at your little one and lets your doctor assess the baby's growth and development. It may also be used to diagnose placental abnormalities, an ectopic pregnancy, certain birth defects or other suspected problems.

There are two types of ultrasound scans: the transabdominal, which scans through your abdomen, and the transvaginal, which scans directly into your vagina. In very early pregnancy, the technician may opt for the vaginal approach, which means that the transducer will be inserted into your vagina. However, abdominal ultrasounds are the most common, as most ultrasounds take place in the second or third trimesters.

An ultrasound typically takes no longer than a half hour to perform. If you are in the first half of your pregnancy, you will probably be instructed to drink plenty of water prior to the exam, and refrain from emptying your bladder. This is probably the most difficult part of the test. The extra fluids help the technician to visualize your baby.

Once in the examining room, you will recline on a table or bed with your upper body elevated and your abdomen exposed. Ask for extra pillows if you tend to get woozy when not lying on your side. The lights may be dimmed to allow the operator to see the sonogram picture more clearly. A thin application of transducer paste, jelly or oil will be spread on your abdomen, and then the fun begins.

I have been offered a nuchal-fold scan. What does this mean?
This is an ultrasound test, done at around 11-14 weeks to measure the fold of skin at the back of the baby's neck. A thicker-than-normal fold could indicate Down's Syndrome. The Nuchal-fold scan does not give a definitive diagnosis, but it is a non-invasive test, and if further investigation is required you may be offered amniocentesis.

The ultrasound picture, or sonogram, is obtained when high-frequency soundwaves are passed over your abdomen with a hand-held wand called a transducer. These waves bounce off the solid structures of your baby, sending back a moving image of the tiny being inside. The resulting picture is transmitted to a computer or television screen. Ultrasound pictures are typically a grainy black and white, but new three-dimensional ultrasound technologies on the market can display your child in living (but simulated) colour and are incredibly lifelike. The two- dimensional units are more common, however, in part because they are much less expensive. Ask the ultrasound operator to print out pictures for you to take home.

The newest wave in ultrasound – four-dimensional technology – is actually 3D with movement added. The picture is clearer, and the movement component allows for diagnosis of heart defects. It can also be used to check for markers of developmentally normal foetal movements.

The ultrasound technician may take a series of measurements during the procedure with the computer attached to the machine. These measurements help your provider assess the growth and organ development of the foetus. Depending on the timing of the test and the cooperation of your unborn child, she may also be able to get an idea of his or her gender. Typically, this information won't be given unless you ask for it, in case you prefer to be surprised at birth. Once the test is over, the technician will help you clean the transducer gel off your belly and you'll be able to empty your bladder, if need be.

When and if you have an ultrasound will depend upon your doctor. Many obstetricians order ultrasounds as a matter of routine. Some do one at the first visit to check for correct dates and viability with the rationale that it may save them from questioning gestational dates later on (as dating is more accurate in the first trimester). Others will recommend a sonogram at around 20 weeks to examine the foetal anatomy and ensure that the pregnancy is progressing normally.

A patient's peace of mind may also be reason enough to order an ultrasound. Since it is a non-invasive and fairly inexpensive test that can reassure the parents that things are developing normally, many doctors will comply with a woman's request for an ultrasound. If your doctor hasn't ordered one and you have some anxieties about your baby's health, it can't hurt to ask.

If your foetus isn't feeling coy on ultrasound day, a sonogram taken after 16 weeks may reveal his or her sex. A sighting of a little girl's labia (visible as three parallel lines) or a boy's penis and testicles is necessary to get a fairly positive ID. As a general rule, your technician will probably not commit herself to an answer on the gender unless she sees one or the other. Just because a penis isn't visible doesn't necessarily mean you have a girl. If you do get a boy or girl answer, keep in mind that barring genetic testing, nothing is 100 per cent certain until you meet the baby after delivery.

Alpha-foetoprotein (AFP)/Triple or Quad Screen Test

Alpha-foetoprotein is a blood protein produced by your unborn baby and passed into your circulatory system. The AFP, administered between weeks 16 and 18, is a blood test used to screen for chromosomal irregularities likespina bifida and Downs syndrome, and also for neural tube defects. Results of this test are usually available in about a week.

Most of the time, a high level of AFP can be explained by multiple gestation (twins, triplets or more). However, it could also mean that your foetus has a neural tube defect. If AFP levels are low, it may be an indication of Downs syndrome or other chromosomal disorders. It could also mean that your dates are wrong. A level-one or level-two ultrasound, or an amniocentesis may be ordered for further evaluation. You may also be referred to a genetic counsellor.

A more extensive version of the AFP, called the triple-screen test (or AFP-3), measures levels of human chorionic gonadotropin (hCG) and oestriol, a type of oestrogen, as well as AFP. The quad-test, an even more sensitive marker of chromosomal problems, assesses all three of these substances plus inhibin-A. The nuchal scan has now replaced this test in many hospitals.

A misdated pregnancy can affect the results of your AFP or triple or quad screen and give a false positive. An ultrasound can help to confirm or adjust the gestational age.

Amniocentesis

The thought of an amniocentesis makes many women nervous, probably because it involves two critical undertakings: a needle being inserted through the abdomen and breaching your baby's watery environment. It does carry some risk of complications, including a slight chance of miscarriage. However, the amnio (as it is commonly referred to) is one of the best tools available for diagnosing chromosomal abnormalities, genetic disorders and birth defects. An amniocentesis is typically performed in the second trimester after week 15 or 16 of pregnancy, although a later amnio may be done, depending on the indication (or reason). At this point in pregnancy there are enough foetal cells present in the amniotic fluid for withdrawal and analysis.

In addition to the wealth of genetic and health information it provides, an amnio can also tell you definitively if your baby is a boy or a girl. If you want to be surprised about the sex of your child, it may be a good idea to restate your wishes before you receive your amnio results.

Your doctor may suggest an appointment with a genetic counsellor prior to having an amniocentesis performed, to weigh the risks versus the benefits of the procedure, given your specific medical background and family history. She will also lay out any alternative procedures that may be options, such as a level-two ultrasound. If you do decide to go with the amnio, you may be sent to a perinatologist, or maternal-foetal specialist, who is experienced in the procedure.

An amniocentesis is a relatively short outpatient procedure. Your abdomen is first swabbed with an antiseptic solution. The physician will use the abdominal ultrasound procedure to see her way around your womb. She will then insert a needle into the amniotic sac and draw an amniotic fluid sample into a syringe. The fluid contains sloughed-off foetal cells, which will be analyzed in the lab.

Here are reasons why an amniocentesis may be planned:

- **Age:** Women over 37 have an increased risk of carrying a baby with a chromosomal disorder like Downs syndrome When the father is over 50, amniocentesis could also be advised because there may be a connection between paternal age and an increased risk of Downs syndrome.
- **Family history:** If you've already had a baby with a hereditary or chromosomal abnormality or neural tube defects, an amniocentesis could make you feel more comfortable.
- **AFP, triple screen or quad-test results:** If alpha-foetoprotein (AFP) shows up at a higher than normal level, an amnio may help clear up any questions.
- **Ultrasound abnormalities:** If your ultrasound turned up indications of the possibility of a chromosomal disorder, an amnio may be recommended for further evaluation.

After the amnio procedure, the baby will be monitored by ultrasound and will have his heart rate checked for a few minutes to ensure that everything is okay. You may experience minimal cramps. You will be advised to restrict strenuous exercise for one day (no step aerobics), although other normal activity should be fine. If in the days following amnio you experience fluid or blood discharge from the vagina, let your doctor know as soon as possible.

There is a slight increase of risk of miscarriage with allm invasive tests. There is also a slight risk of trauma to the unborn baby from a misplaced needle or inadvertent rupture of the sac.

If there are problems, the information you get from an amnio can prepare you for providing your child with the best care possible at birth. However, the timing can make other decisions difficult. Results from your amniocentesis won't be available for up to two weeks. And by the time the test results are back, you will be halfway through your pregnancy (about 20 weeks). For this reason, some women at risk for chromosomal abnormalities will choose the chorionic villus sampling test, which can be performed in the first trimester, instead.

Chorionic Villus Sampling (CVS)

CVS stands for chorionic villus sampling, a test performed in the first trimester (usually between weeks 10 and 12) to assess chromosomal abnormalities and hereditary conditions in the unborn baby. Your provider will use ultrasound guidance to insert a catheter into the placenta, either through the cervix (transcervical) or through a needle injected into the abdomen (transabdominal). The catheter is used to extract a biopsy (or sample) of the tiny chorionic villi, the fingers of tissue surrounding the embryo that are the beginnings of the placenta. The villi are a genetic match for the baby's own tissue.

Slight cramp and spotting are normal after the procedure, and you will probably be advised to indulge in some rest and relaxation for the remainder of the day. If bleeding continues, is excessive or is accompanied by pain or fever, call your doctor immediately.

CVS has several benefits over amnio. It can be performed earlier (first trimester as opposed to second), and the results are available much faster (5–7 days for preliminary CVS results versus 10–14 days for amnio). However, the risk of miscarriage is about 1 per cent higher than the spontaneous miscarriage rate. The risk is higher for woman with a retroverted (tipped, or tilted) uterus who are given a transcervical CVS. For this reason, a transabdominal CVS (through the abdominal wall) is usually advised for these women. An appointment with a genetic counsellor can help you analyze the positives and negatives and decide if a CVS is right for you.

A CVS is not always accurate. The exact spot where the technician removes the cell sampling from the chorion can be critical. Also, some abnormalities in chorionic tissues do not always show up in the foetus. Ask for clarification or a second opinion of any negative CVS report before you decide on any course of action in your pregnancy.

Foetal Monitoring

A foetal heart monitor measures – you guessed it – the foetal heart rate (or FHR). A baseline, or average, foetal heart rate of 120–160 beats per minute (bpm) is considered normal. Spikes as high as 25 bpm are normal and coincide with foetal stimulation and sleep cycles.

During Labour

Foetal monitors also measure the length and severity of contractions. There are both external and internal monitors available. An external monitor uses two belts that are positioned around your belly. The transducers on each are adjusted until they are both measuring your contractions and picking up the foetal heart sounds.

If you are in a high-risk pregnancy, you may be hooked up to an internal foetal monitor during labour and delivery. Internal monitors may only be used in labour when the amniotic sac has broken. This monitor is considered more sensitive and accurate, but is also more invasive. It uses a little spring-like wire that is inserted vaginally and sits just under the skin on the baby's head.

Both internal and external monitoring can keep you tethered to your bed during labour, which may not be the experience you want. External monitors, however, can be removed for a short time, but in general foetal movement should be assessed at least every 15 minutes. A new type of monitor, which uses telemetry, allows some women to go wireless for labour. For more on telemetry, see Chapter 18.

Chapter 6

Month 3

This is a landmark month as you finish up your first trimester! You start to sport a protruding belly, which may mean sharing your news with friends, family and colleagues, if you haven't already. Your little foetus is growing by leaps and bounds, and you make first contact this month as you hear her heartbeat and perhaps even see her on ultrasound.

Baby This Month

By the end of this month, baby will grow to over 75mm (3in) in length and almost 30g (1oz). If you could look at his face, you'd see that his ears and closed eyelids have now fully developed. His head accounts for one-third of his total length, and his tongue, salivary glands and taste buds have also formed. Even though he's a long way from his first meal, studies indicate he may already be getting a taste of what you've been snacking on from the maternal blood supply or placenta.

He is now getting all of his nutrients through the fully formed placenta (from the Greek *plakous*, meaning flat cake, its approximately shape), an organ that you and your foetus share. The umbilical cord tethers the foetus to the placenta, which provides it with nutrients and oxygen and transports waste materials away.

Your baby's heart is pumping about 27 litres of blood each day, and a lattice of blood vessels can be seen through his translucent skin, which is starting to develop a coat of fine, downy hair called lanugo. His or her gender is apparent since the external sex organs have now fully differentiated, but it will take a combination of luck and technical skill for an ultrasound operator to reveal if you have a son or daughter. (For more on ultrasound exams, see Chapter 5.)

While the greatest risk of miscarriage is in the first trimester, by the time you hear your baby's heartbeat around week 12, the placenta has fully formed and the risk of miscarriage has dropped significantly.

Your Body This Month

You probably never thought you'd be pleased by a potbellied profile, but this significant, visible sign of your pregnancy is a landmark moment for many women. Wear it proudly. You've taken your child through the first three critical months of growth, and your belly is a badge of honour that tells the world about this important accomplishment.

Your Body Changes

Your uterus now stretches to just about your pubic bone. About 0.9–1.8kg (2–4lb) total weight gain is average for the first trimester; if you've been down and out with nausea and vomiting, you may be below the curve. Weight gain will pick up in the second trimester and peak in the third as your baby starts to fill out your womb.

▲ You and your foetus at the end of the first trimester.

Don't take the 'eating for two' cliché literally – 300 extra calories per day is about all you'll require to meet your baby's nutritional needs.

Gaining too much can exacerbate the aches and pains of pregnancy, place an extra strain on your back, and may put you at risk for hypertension (high blood pressure) problems.

At the same time, if you find the aversions and nausea of pregnancy mean you can only keep down a certain type of not-so-nutritious food (pepperoni pizza, for example), don't feel bad about it. The most important thing right now is keeping food down and your energy up. Try experimenting with some healthier variations if your stomach will take it (skip the pepperoni in exchange for extra cheese or vegetables), and hang on in there. By the end of the first trimester most women report that their morning sickness gets better or (fingers crossed) completely disappears.

While 10–15kg (25–35lb) is the average suggested total weight gain for a pregnancy, your height and build will influence that number. Underweight women and women with multiple pregnancies (twins or more) will be expected to gain more, overweight women will be encouraged to gain slightly less. If your doctor hasn't mentioned a weight goal for your pregnancy, ask him what his expectations are.

Most important, don't let the scale become an obsession. Focus instead on the quality of food you're eating and on getting some regular exercise (cleared with your doctor first). Your health and baby's health are the ultimate goals of this pregnancy.

Breakdown of where the weight goes
Baby – 3.4–3.8kg (7.5–8.5lb)
Uterus – 0.9–1.1kg (2–2.5lb)

Breakdown of where the weight goes *(cont'd)*
Placenta – 0.72–0.9kg (1.5–2lb)
Amniotic fluid – (0.9kg (2lb)
Blood – 1.3–1.8kg (3–4lb)
Breasts – 0.45–0.9kg (1–2lb)
Maternal fat and nutrient stores – 1.8–2.7kg (4–6lb)
Retained maternal fluids – 1.8–3.6kg (4–8lb)

What You Feel Like

Although nausea and vomiting may finally be waning, thanks to a decline in hCG levels, constipation, wind and occasional heartburn may take over as the gastrointestinal pests of the next trimester. Constipation is caused by an increase in progesterone, which can act to slow down the digestive system. Later in the pregnancy, pressure on the intestine caused by your growing uterus adds to the problem.

An increase in dietary fibre, plenty of water intake and exercise, as approved by your caregiver or doctor, may also help to get things going again. Make sure you consult your doctor before taking any stool softeners or laxatives.

Wind may become a source of discomfort and occasional embarrassment as well. Consider cutting back on foods that worsen the problem (e.g. onions, beans, broccoli, cabbage, carbonated drinks). Fibre you take to eliminate constipation can also aggravate wind problems. Try small, frequent snacks instead of large meals to keep the burps at bay.

Other pregnancy symptoms that may continue or begin this month include:

- Fatigue
- Frequent urination
- Tender breasts
- Nausea

- Headaches
- Increased saliva
- Nasal congestion and/or runny nose
- Occasional dizziness or faintness

At the Doctor

Make sure your husband or partner makes this month's prenatal appointment. You're both in for a treat as you begin to experience the sights and sounds of your growing child.

Tests This Month

Depending on your doctor's policy on ultrasound exams and your personal medical history, you may be seeing your baby this month. For the complete story on ultrasound examinations, see Chapter 5.

Your doctor will also start estimating the size of your baby by taking a tape measure to your belly and counting the centimetres from your pubic bone to the tip of your fundus – the top of the uterus. Taking this measurement at each visit gives your doctor a way to assess your baby's ongoing growth. Some doctors do not take the fundal height until after week 12 or even week 20.

Fundal height is used as a screening tool only; women who are overweight, carrying multiples or have a foetus in the breech position may not measure accurately.

Baby's Heartbeat

Hearing the steady 'woosh-woosh' of your baby's heart for the first time is one of the most thrilling and emotional moments of pregnancy. Your chance at first contact happens this month as your provider checks for the foetal heartbeat using a small ultrasound device called a Doppler or Doptone. If you have a retroverted uterus (also known as a tipped or tilted uterus), it's possible the Doppler won't detect the heartbeat just yet. Don't be alarmed; by your next prenatal appointment you will probably be able to hear her loud and clear.

I've reached the magic 15-week mark and I'm still sick as a dog. Could I be having twins?
While lingering and/or excessive nausea and vomiting in pregnancy can indicate twins, in the absence of other signs of multiples it's more likely a simple matter of your unique body chemistry and pregnancy. Hang on in there, talk to your doctor, and try some of the morning sickness suggestions in Chapter 2. (Also see Chapter 7.)

On Your Mind

Feel like you're losing your mind while gaining three dress sizes? Coping with forgetfulness and learning to love your changing body are just a few of the issues facing you as you get to the close of the first trimester.

Forgetfulness

Have you walked around looking for your sunglasses for 20 minutes before finding them on your head? Lost your car keys for the fifth time this week? Like any mum-to-be, you've got a lot on your mind. That alone may have you forgetting what used to be second nature and misplacing things. Although researchers have looked at the problem of memory impairment in pregnancy, there hasn't been a clear consensus on what the definitive cause is.

Pregnancy hormones, sleep deprivation and stress have all been suggested as possible culprits. A 2002 study published in the *Journal of Reproductive Medicine* found that women in their second trimester of pregnancy who reported memory problems had lower blood levels of the neurotransmitters norepinephrine, epinephrine and serotonin than their non-pregnant peers, suggesting that these brain chemicals may somehow be related to memory loss.

Whatever the cause, forgetting appointments and misplacing things can leave you feeling muddled and helpless. Try relying less on your memory by writing notes, sticking to a routine (e.g. car keys always go into a basket by the door), and living by a written or electronic organizer. If you aren't the Palm Pilot type, start requesting a 24-hour advance phone call reminder when you schedule service appointments such as in-home appliance repair or a salon appointment. Having a system – whatever it is – is the key to staying reasonably organized and mentally together during this hectic time.

Feeling Good about Your Changing Body

A word about weight – try not to get too hung up on it. Stepping on the scale at every doctor's visit may make weight seem like a pass or fail test, but it is just one tool your provider has to make sure your baby is growing on schedule. Don't dread the regular weigh-in – look at what it tells you as tangible proof your unborn child is growing and developing well.

Never diet in pregnancy, even if you've already gained more than expected. Restricting calorie and nutrient intake can hamper foetal development. If you're concerned about excessive weight gain, consider seeing a registered dietitian for help with meal planning and/or taking an approved prenatal exercise class.

Don't compare yourself to those who have gone before you, either. If older neighbours, friends and relatives remark on their own minimal weight gain and quick return to pre-pregnancy weight, there's a reason for this. Up to and including the 1970s, 'ideal' pregnancy weight gains averaged 4–6.2kg (10–15lb) less than they do today, according to the Institute of Medicine. Further studies have since shown that weight gain should be individualized to a mother's pre-pregnancy body mass index (BMI), and that inadequate weight gain can actually contribute to low-birthweight babies.

Now is a good time to go out and buy that first maternity outfit if you haven't already done so. Pick out something comfortable and stylish that makes you feel good, and maybe even shows off your belly a bit.

Spreading the Word

Now that you're showing, keeping your pregnancy to yourself will be increasingly difficult. If you and your partner have kept the good news to yourself so far – for a whole trimester, no less – now is probably the time to spill the beans.

Sharing with Friends and Family

How you tell your parents, siblings and best friends that you and your partner are pregnant can be one of the most exciting parts of pregnancy. It can also be a little nerve-racking if you're not sure how your news will be received.

If you've held off sharing your pregnancy until now, 'Why did you wait so long to tell us?' may be a common refrain. Whatever your reasons for waiting are, they're valid. Let your family and friends know that they're important to you, which is why you've chosen to make them among the first outside of you and your partner to know about your new addition.

Some fun ideas for sharing the news with parents, friends or others:

- Give them an ultrasound picture (or a photocopy of one), and let it explain itself.
- Send out birthday invitations for the estimated due date.
- Take out a 'Help Wanted: Grandparents' advertisement in their local classifieds and point it out to them to the grandparents.
- If this isn't your first, let your kids spread the news in their own special way.
- The old standby – 'Guess what?' – works well, too.

Alas, there are some people in the world who are perpetually in the glass-half-empty state of mind. You may be related to one of them. If you expect a negative reaction from someone who must be clued in on the pregnancy (read: immediate family member), try to take along your spouse or partner for emotional support. Hopefully, the wet blanket will surprise you both with a hug and well wishes. If not, treat yourself to a date with your partner and let it go as a character defect – theirs.

When (and What) to Tell Work

Now that your pregnancy is becoming more visible and your doctor's appointments are taking you away from the office on a regular basis, it may be a good time to let your employer in on your secret. From a practical viewpoint, you'll want to find out about your company's leave policy, maternity benefits, and health insurance coverage for new family members.

So how do you break the news? Make sure you tell your supervisor or manager first. Hearing about your impending maternity leave through the grapevine may make your manager question your future commitment to your career. Go into the meeting with an idea of how much maternity leave you'd like to take and, even better, who might cover your job responsibilities while you're away.

If you're asked about your plans after baby is born, be honest while playing your cards close to your vest. If you're happy with your career and workplace but unsure whether your tune will change once you see your darling son or daughter, let your employer know you have every intention of returning to work and leave it at that. Disingenuous? Not at all. You can't give a definite response on something that hasn't even occurred yet. That's like asking your employer to make a hiring decision on an applicant he hasn't interviewed yet. You can, however, give him your assurances that you're pleased with your position, if that's the case.

On the other hand, if you've already decided that motherhood will be your new full-time vocation, leaving right after your maternity leave runs out, with no fair warning to your supervisor, is a guaranteed way to burn your bridges and ruin your references.

Check your partner's health insurance and see if you can be switched over to it now, so you can give your employer ample notice to find a replacement. If you're worried about losing your job before you're ready to go, let your supervisor or superior know for how long you'd like to work, and don't forget to point out the advantages of using the time to have you train your replacement.

For more on working through and beyond pregnancy, see Chapter 9.

Just for Dads

A boy to bond with or a girl to graduate with honours from Oxford? You and your partner may be thinking about the prospect of a son or daughter, especially if you have an ultrasound appointment approaching. If you're going to try and find out the gender of your child, keep an open mind since you have little choice in the matter. Think instead of the exceptional beauties and joys to be found in both sexes, and the special sibling relationships to be forged, both between and among brothers and sisters. More importantly, start thinking of your baby in terms of potential rather than gender-imposed limitations – girls can carry on the family name just as readily as boys.

Speaking of names, you have probably already started to think about names for the little one. Below are the most popular names for babies born in 2003.

The 10 most popular U.S. baby names for 2002			
Boys' Names		**Girls' Names**	
1. Jack	6. Oliver	1. Emily	6. Megan
2. Joshua	7. Benjamin	2. Ellie	7. Lucy
3. Thomas	8. Samuel	3. Chloe	8. Olivia
4. James	9. William	4. Jessica	9. Charlotte
5. Daniel	10. Joseph	5. Sophie	10. Hannah

The Cost of Kids

Worried about how to make ends meet as your family grows? First, read our Chapter 3 tips on financial planning and paying for pregnancy. Then, sit down with your partner and work through a budget together. The chances are that there's a lot of room for cutting back, and a lot of things – such as films, concerts and those weekend breaks – that you won't be doing, or paying for, any more (at least until your child is a little older).

Still concerned that you won't bring home enough to support your family? You might look at pregnancy as a new beginning for you as well. If you've been thinking about making a career move, brush up your CV and get networking now while things are still relatively quiet in your household. Even if you really love your job, finding out what else is out there and getting an offer on the table can give you leverage for negotiating with your current employer.

Changing Roles

You, a dad? The same guy whose idea of a savings account is six months' worth of change in a water cooler bottle? The same guy who still collects *Star Wars* action figures ('Ahem – that's *collectables*')? The same guy who still calls his dad when the car acts up, and who has 20 more years of student loan repayment ahead of him? It's hard to grasp until you actually experience it, but the responsibilities, intense love and fierce protectiveness that are part of parenthood will make you feel more 'adult' than just about any event in your life thus far. Believe it or not, some day that little boy or girl will be calling you for automotive advice (and playing with your collectables).

Chapter 7

Multiple Choice: Two, Three, Four or More

News of impending twins, triplets and other multiple gestations is certainly a thrilling, and momentous, surprise for any couple. Disbelief, distinction and panic are just a few of the feelings you might experience on the road to a multiple birth.

Splitting Eggs and Sharing Sacs

Multiples are either monozygotic (formed from a single egg and sperm) or dizygotic (formed from two separate eggs and sperm). Monozygotic multiples, more commonly known as 'identicals', can be further classified by the way they share their common space and maternal resources.

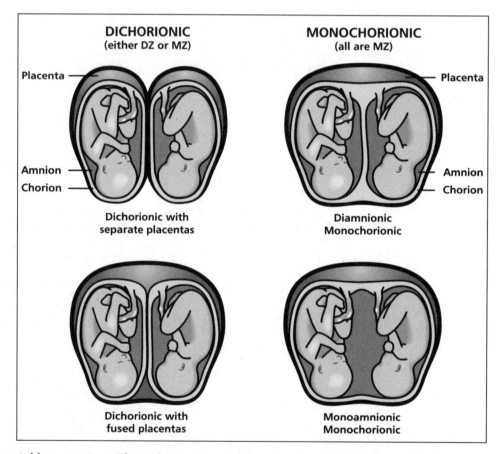

DICHORIONIC
(either DZ or MZ)

MONOCHORIONIC
(all are MZ)

Placenta

Placenta

Amnion

Amnion

Chorion

Chorion

Dichorionic with separate placentas

Diamnionic Monochorionic

Dichorionic with fused placentas

Monoamnionic Monochorionic

▲ Monozygotic, or identical, twins may each have its own set of foetal membranes, or they may share an amniotic sac (monoamniotic), a chorion membrane (monochorionic), or both.

Identical Twins

Identical, or monozygotic, twins form when a single fertilized egg (zygote) splits in two. Because they are cut from the same piece of genetic fabric, they are always the same gender. Monozygotic twins also share a placenta. Depending on when the zygote splits, they may share an amniotic sac and/or the chorionic membrane, or they may each have their own personal space and membranes. Twins that split more than a week after fertilization will probably share both the amnion and the chorion, while twins that split early on are more likely to have separate quarters.

A single zygote that produces twins usually splits within days of fertilization, but may wait up to two weeks. Zygotes that split beyond 14 days increase the risk of resulting in conjoined twins, or twins who haven't separated completely and develop with shared body parts or organ systems. Fraternal twins, because they start life as two eggs fertilized by two sperms, do not run the risk of conjoinment.

Fraternal Multiples

Fraternal, or dizygotic, twins are basically siblings in the womb. Each one is created from a separate egg fertilized with its own sperm. Fraternal twins are three times more common than identical twins. They have their own placentas, can be the same or different genders, and may not look any more alike than siblings born individually.

Who Has Multiple Births?

Your chances of having twins are actually not that big – about 1 in 90 births result in twins. If fraternal twins run in your family, your odds are slightly higher. The number of twins and multiple births has skyrocketed over the past several decades, mainly as a result of fertility treatments which stimulate the ovaries, or procedures such as IVF, where more than one embryo is implanted.

Statistics also reveal that more women are waiting until their thirties and forties to have children, and the increasing twin rate may reflect that reality. Women over 35, especially those who have had a previous multiple birth, have an increased chance of having multiples.

While birth outcomes of a singleton pregnancy involve more risk as maternal age increases, researchers at the National Institute of Child Health and Human Development (NICHD) and University of Kansas have found that the opposite seems to hold true for multiples pregnancies among older mums. In fact, their 2002 study comparing birth outcomes in triplet pregnancies found that mums over 35 had healthier babies with fewer complications than younger triplet moms. This is probably due in part to the increased use of IVF in older women, and the fact that IVF multiples rarely share the same amniotic sac — a risk factor for a number of prenatal complications in multiple pregnancies.

Your Body in Multiples Pregnancy

You are living larger than you ever imagined. With all those arms and legs flailing about, you feel as if you're housing a team of tiny Olympic hopefuls. Although it may not feel like it when your crowd is going wild and your back is killing you, a multiple pregnancy is a truly unique gift. That your body can accommodate and nurture not just one, but two, three or possibly more human beings is nothing short of miraculous.

Mums-to-be of multiples experience the same pregnancy symptoms as women with only one foetus, but they may be more intense and occur earlier in the pregnancy. Excessive nausea and vomiting, in particular, is often an early sign that your unborn child has company. However, many women with single pregnancies can experience severe morning sickness as well. More significant markers of multiple pregnancies would include the presence of more than one foetal heart tone during a prenatal examination and measuring too large for your suspected gestational age after week 24.

High levels of alpha-foetoprotein (AFP) on an AFP, triple-screen or quad-screen blood test may also be an indication that you have some stowaways. For more on AFP, see Chapter 5.

Doctor's Visits

If you've been diagnosed with a multiple pregnancy, you'll be visiting your doctor more frequently. Your appointment schedule will depend on your specific medical history and risk factors involved with your pregnancy, but your cartegivers will want to see you more often.

Diagnosis

While a number of symptoms and screening tests may point to a multiple pregnancy, a definitive diagnosis is usually made by ultrasound. During the ultrasound procedure, the technician will try to determine whether or not the foetuses are sharing a single amniotic sac, since this may put them at higher risk for some complications.

Other mums of twins or multiples can be a great source of information, support and advice for the unique issues you face, both during pregnancy and after birth. You don't have to stake out the local parks looking for twins; a local or regional 'parents of multiples club' can put you in touch with someone in your area. Contact the Twins and Multiple Births Association at www.tamba.org.uk.

Problems in Multiple Pregnancies

Multiple pregnancies have a shorter gestation time than single pregnancies, simply because there just aren't enough room and resources in mum to house the brood for 40 weeks. Full term for a twin pregnancy is considered 38 weeks (triplets are full term at 35 weeks and quads at 34 weeks). The biggest risk by far in a multiple pregnancy is preterm labour and premature birth.

Problems Mum May Face

If your body is nourishing two or more children, you need to treat it with a little extra TLC. Take an additional 600 calories daily of healthy foods (beyond average prepregnancy calorie intake), and drink plenty of water.

The latter is particularly important, since dehydration can trigger off preterm contractions.

Although due dates are typically based on a ten-lunar-month calendar, most people consider pregnancy a nine-month, three-trimester affair. That's why you'll find your pregnancy divided into nine calendar months in this book. (For more on estimating your due date, see Chapter 2.)

Mums-to-be of multiples are at greater risk of developing anaemia, and should speak to their doctor about iron supplements to ensure that their needs are covered. Increasing your intake of iron-rich foods is a good way to ward off anaemia: try rotating iron-fortified foods, such as baked beans, blackstrap molasses, wheatgerm, raisins, beef and leafy green vegetables (spinach, kale and broccoli into your diet. For more on eating correctly in pregnancy, see Chapter 1.

The cervix has heavy work to do in a multiple pregnancy. Even the simple act of standing has gravity working against you. In women with a short cervix (approximately 25mm/1in or less at 24 weeks), some reinforcements may be required. If cervical incompetence is suspected, a transvaginal ultrasound, in which the Doppler wand is inserted into the vagina rather than moved across the belly, is used to assess cervical length and monitor the progress of the cervix. As a preventative measure, your provider may suggest a cerclage – a procedure involving suturing (or stitching) the cervix closed to avoid preterm dilation. Studies are inconclusive as to whether or not cervical cerclage is effective in improving birth outcomes, but it does appear that the earlier cerclage is performed in the pregnancy, the more potential it has for success. Cerclage is usually performed in the second trimester.

Almost half of all multiple pregnancies result in preterm labour (labour before 37 weeks). If you start having contractions or other signs of preterm labour and are still less than 4cm (1³/8in) dilated, your provider may try to halt labour until you're further along in your pregnancy, using one or more of the following methods:

- **Bed rest:** Strict bed rest may be imposed to keep the pressure off your cervix. This could be at home (with a few toilet visits granted) or in a hospital. A foetal monitor may be used to keep an eye on the team's progress.
- **Fluids:** You may be hooked up to an intravenous line and/or fed fluids to keep you hydrated.
- **Trendelenburg position:** Bed rest – to the extreme. If your doctor mentions this, he wants you on a bed that works against gravity by elevating your feet and tilting your head down.
- **Tocolytic medication:** Tocolytic drugs, such as magnesium sulfate, calcium channel blockers and terbutaline may be administered by mouth or intravenously to stop contractions.
- **Antibiotics:** If your membranes have ruptured prematurely (preterm premature rupture of membranes, or PPROM), antibiotics can help to ward off infection. They are also used to prevent group B strep infection of the preterm newborn.

There are some situations where tocolysis should not be attempted, even if you are considerably preterm. If monitoring indicates that your foetus is in distress, if you have signs of infection of the amniotic fluid, if you are bleeding excessively or if you are pre-eclamptic, tocolyctic drugs are not recommended. In most of these cases, immediate delivery by Caesarean section will be required.

Problems Babies May Face

Up to 70 per cent of monoamniotic twins and higher-order multiples experience umbilical cord knotting, twisting or entanglement. In severe cases, kinks or tangles in the cord can cut off blood supply to one or both foetuses. Ultrasound can determine the presence or absence of a dividing membrane between multiples. If a multiple monoamniotic pregnancy is detected, it will be followed closely with routine ultrasounds to check for umbilical cord complications.

Twin-to-twin transfusion syndrome (TTTS) is a rare condition affecting approximately 10 per cent of those 'identical' twins who share a chorionic membrane and placenta. In TTTS, an abnormality in the placenta causes irregularities in foetal blood circulation, and blood is shunted between the foetuses through placental vessels that connect them. The result is that one foetus experiences cardiovascular overload and potential heart failure, while the other receives insufficient blood flow. TTTS is not limited to twins, and can occur in higher-order multiple pregnancies as well.

A laser-surgical technique developed in the 1980s can be used to successfully treat some cases of TTTS. Foetoscopic laser occlusion of the connecting placental blood vessels (FLOC) uses an endoscope (a thin, flexible tube with a tiny camera attached) to find the blood vessels connecting multiples and close them off.

In addition to its involvement with TTTS, the position and construction of the placenta can impact the growth of one or more multiples. Maternal blood flow and nutrition may be unequally distributed among foetuses, resulting in an uneven growth rate among them. Multiples are also at a higher risk for intrauterine growth retardation (IUGR). For more on that condition, see Chapter 13.

Vanishing twin syndrome is the death of one twin that was previously viable. When it occurs early in pregnancy, the body is typically reabsorbed into the uterine wall. Some minor bleeding and cramp may signal the process. More serious complications may result if vanishing twin syndrome happens later in pregnancy.

Other conditions multiples are considered at high risk for include congenital abnormalities and placental problems (e.g. placenta previa, placental abruption). For more on these conditions, see Chapter 13.

Delivering Multiples

Nothing is routine in a multiple pregnancy, and the surprises will likely keep coming through labour and delivery as well.

Caesarean versus Vaginal Delivery

About half of all twins are born via Caesarean section, and the number goes up considerably for triplets or more. Because of the risk of umbilical cord entanglement, multiples that share an amniotic sac are usually delivered by Caesarean at or before 34 weeks.

Whether other multiples are delivered vaginally or not will depend on how they are positioned in the womb. If the first baby is breech (feet or buttocks first), your provider will probably prefer Caesarean. If at least the first baby is vertex (head down), a vaginal delivery may be performed. Women who feel strongly about having a vaginal delivery of their multiples should talk to their doctor early on in the pregnancy about the issue.

A quick ultrasound in the labour and delivery room will reveal your babies' positions. In some cases, external cephalic version may be attempted to turn a stubborn twin (for more on version, see Chapter 16). In most cases of twin vaginal birth, the provider will attempt to deliver the second baby within 15 minutes of the first, to minimize possible complications.

Premature Birth

Babies who are born prematurely are at risk of respiratory distress syndrome (RDS) due to lung immaturity.

Postpartum Haemorrhage

Women who have delivered multiples are at an increased risk for postpartum haemorrhage, or excessive bleeding, after delivery. Some of the tocolyctic medications (e.g. magnesium sulfate) can also increase the risk of bleeding by inhibiting uterine muscle function. Once the placenta is delivered, the uterus must continue to contract in order to tamp down and seal off placental blood vessels. In a womb that is overstretched from multiples, the myometrium – the smooth muscle layer responsible for contractions – may not function efficiently. Postpartum haemorrhage can be the result.

If postpartum haemorrhage does occur, the uterus will be double-checked for any remaining pieces of the placenta (another cause of postpartum bleeding) and massaged to control the bleeding. Oxytocin or prostaglandin may also be administered to stimulate contractions.

When Babies Are in Intensive Care

You've waited and waited to hold your babies in your arms, and now they're in the neonatal intensive care unit, behind glass and bound up by wires and tubes. Be assured that even though they may be dependent on machines, your presence and parental touch are critical in speeding their recovery and eventual discharge.

'Kangaroo care', skin-to-skin parent-and-premature contact, has been shown to have a positive impact on parent-child bonding and improve the motor and cognitive development of premature babies. But early on, some very premature babies may not yet be ready for the sensory overload of touching. Be assured that they will want and need it as time goes on, and staff and neonatal physiotherapists can instruct you on methods of nurturing forms of touch for your children.

Never forget that your presence is essential to making this scary, sterile world a loving, temporary home for your children. Holding their tiny hands, getting involved with their care and feeding, and learning how to care for any unique medical needs are all critical tasks right now. The skilled nursing staff can be a tremendous resource as you get comfortable with your children's care. Tap into their expertise while you have the opportunity.

Barring any other serious medical problems, your new family members will be discharged from the hospital once they've reached a predetermined weight goal (usually around 2kg/4.4 lb) and are able to maintain their body temperature and feed and breathe well on their own. If any of your children require special medical monitoring or attention after discharge, home visits from a nurse can help you get adjusted to their care routine. Turn to Chapter 13 for more on preterm birth.

Surviving the First Month Home

Be it hired help, grandparents or friends, you absolutely must have backup support when you're bringing home multiples. Ideally, you'll organize your recruits well before birth, but this isn't always possible given the unpredictability of due dates with multiples. Think about designating a trusted friend or relative to delegate tasks – someone who's organized and dependable. Try not to lumber your partner with the job; both of you will have your hands full when the kids are finally here.

Schedules, Schedules, Schedules

Depending on the number of babies you're juggling, and whether you're breast- or bottle-feeding, it may seem easier at first to just feed them all on demand. However, that strategy may eventually be at the expense of sleep and sanity. Without a little help, they will continue to follow their own timetable, the one that has you grabbing sleep in 20-minute bits.

So how do you get your little ones into the programme? A rigid feeding and sleep schedule is doomed to failure; newborns need to know you're there for them, no matter what the agenda says. A more practical and flexible approach is to wake up all the babies once one wakes up to eat. Feeding them all simultaneously and then laying them back down to sleep will get them on track toward a feeding schedule that's more or less in synch.

Your babies will probably not sleep longer than two hours at a stretch to start, so having them in your bedroom or getting a comfortable bedroll or inflatable mattress for the nursery floor may be a good idea for those nights when even finding your way back to bed seems too time-intensive.

Breast, Bottle or Both?

The moment you hear 'multiples', breast-feeding takes on a whole new dimension. Visions of becoming a 24-hour, all-you-can-eat buffet for this litter of babies may have you revisiting your plans to nurse exclusively. Before you make any rash decisions, know that mothers of multiples can and do breast-feed (and live to tell about it!).

At the same time, don't let anyone tell you that it will be easy. It will take a lot of hard work and persistence – and an equal amount of support from family and friends – to nurse your babies successfully. But the health, bonding and cost benefits can make it well worth your while.

Why breast-feed your brood? First of all, breast milk is cheaper and more convenient for a single baby; multiply that time and money savings by two or more and you end up with quite a deal. In addition, multiples may get an even bigger immunity boost from breast milk because of their tendency to be preterm and low birth weight babies, two factors that raise their risk for other health problems. And breast-feeding provides special one-on-one time with each child.

Many mums of twins find that nursing both children at once (tandem nursing) is the most efficient way of taking care of feeding time. This may be a little tricky at the onset, but you'll get better with practice. An appointment with a lactation consultant is a good idea for breast-feeding mothers of multiples to get pointers on scheduling, logistics and more.

Football hold

◄ Mothers of multiples can nurse two babies simultaneously in a number of positions – including the football, parallel, crisscross, and front V holds.

Parallel hold

Crisscross hold

Front V hold

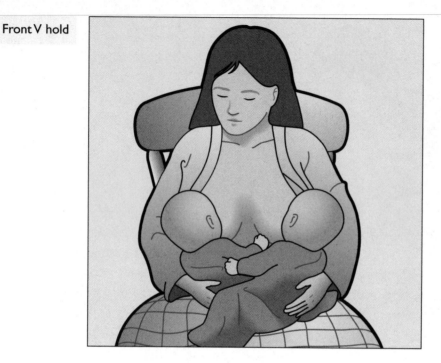

Bottle-feeding can have its positive side as well, particularly with higher-order multiples. The biggest benefit is that your partner or other helpers can get in on the action, a huge plus if you're trying to get two or more on the same feeding and sleeping schedule. And if you have an impatient eater in your crew, you don't have to worry about making him wait his turn while the others nurse.

Really want to provide your children with the health benefits of breast milk, but finding the physical toll of nursing multiples overwhelming? Some women choose to rotate a formula feeding among their multiples while the others feed at the breast. However, this may result in a diminished milk supply over time. Consider augmenting a few breast-feedings a day with a bottle filled with pumped milk instead. For more on breast-feeding, see Chapter 19.

Chapter 8

Month 4

Welcome to the second trimester, or what many women consider 'the fun part'. Your energy is up, and your meals are staying down. You and your baby are heading into a period of rapid growth now, so hang on and enjoy the ride. Here's a look at what you can look forward to in month 4.

Baby This Month

Snoozing, stretching, swallowing and even thumb-sucking, your foetus is busy this month as he tests out his new reflexes and abilities. He is losing his top-heavy look as his height starts to catch up to his head size. By the end of this month, he will measure about 15–20cm (6–8in) in length and weigh approximately 175g (6oz).

▲ You and your foetus in month 4 of pregnancy.

Now is a good time to begin singing, reading and even playing music for your little one. The inner ear structures that allow him to hear are developing this month (for more on foetal hearing, see Chapter 12). He has grown eyebrows, eyelashes and possibly even a little hair up on top.

The long bones of his arms and legs are growing as cartilage is replaced with spongy, woven soft bone in a process called ossification. Skeletal development will continue long after birth and well into adolescence and young adulthood.

Your baby is inhaling and exhaling amniotic fluid, practising his technique for his first breath in the outside world. The lungs are already generating cellular fluid and a substance known as surfactant. In later months the surfactant will assist the development of the foetal lungs by expanding the alveoli, or air sacs, within them. These substances move out through the trachea and become part of the amniotic fluid, along with the urine your unborn child is already passing.

f@ct

The umbilical cord contains two arteries and a vein sheathed with a gelatinous tissue known as Wharton's jelly. The jelly cushions the blood vessels and protects them from kinks and twists. Although umbilical cord knots do occur, they are relatively rare, happening in approximately 1 per cent of pregnancies.

The placenta is approximately 75mm (3in) in diameter this month, and the attached umbilical cord is about as long as the foetus and continues to grow. Foetal blood is being pumped through this little body at about 4 miles an hour, exiting through two large arteries in the umbilical cord and on to the placenta. In the placenta, baby's waste products (urine and carbon dioxide) are exchanged for oxygenated, nutrient-rich blood that is returned to the foetus via an umbilical cord vein. Pressure from the blood pumping within the cord helps straighten it out and keeps it from becoming knotted or getting in the way of your unborn baby's kicks and somersaults. Total time for this complex exchange? About 30 seconds.

Your Body This Month

In pregnancy, feeling is believing. While hearing baby's heartbeat or seeing foetal movement on an ultrasound monitor are milestone moments, the first time you actually sense your child inside you – proof positive that you are indeed nurturing an actual human being – is a humbling and life-affirming experience.

Your Body Changes

If you weren't showing last month, chances are you will have a definite pregnant profile by the end of this month. Your uterus is about the size of a head of cabbage, and its top tip lies just below your belly button.

> The thin line of fine hair that runs from your navel down to your pubic bone – the *linea alba* – may turn dark in pregnancy again thanks to hormonal changes. If you do develop this little stripe, now called a *linea nigra*, it will most likely lighten again postpartum.

What You Feel Like

Your appetite may start to pick up this month, especially if you've been too sick to enjoy a good meal until now. You'll need a healthy craving or two to fuel foetal growth – about 60 per cent of your total pregnancy weight (about 5–6.75kg/11–15lb) will be gained in this trimester. (For more on weight gain in pregnancy, see Chapter 6.)

Heartburn may start to become a persistent problem as your uterus crowds your stomach and the smooth muscles of your digestive tract remain relaxed from the hormone progesterone. Some tips for putting out the fire:

·   Avoid greasy, fatty and spicy foods.
·   Stay away from alcohol and caffeinated drinks (e.g. cola, tea, coffee); these may relax the valve between the stomach and the esophagus and exacerbate heartburn.
·   Keep a food log to try to determine what your heartburn triggers are.
·   Eat smaller, more frequent meals instead of three large ones.
·   Drink plenty of water *between* meals to reduce stomach acid.
·   Don't eat just before you go to bed or lie down to rest.

· Pile a few extra pillows on the bed to assist gravity in easing heartburn while you sleep.

If heartburn symptoms won't relent, have a talk with your doctor to find out what can be done.

Calcium – it does a baby good. Your little one needs lots of calcium to build bone and blood cells, and if she doesn't get it in your diet, she'll draw on your skeletal storehouse instead. Milk is an excellent source; four 250ml (8fl oz) glasses daily will provide you with the recommended 1,200mg. Yogurt, broccoli, kale and salmon are rich in calcium as well.

As if heartburn wasn't enough to deal with, pregnancy may start to become a real pain in the rear, literally. Many women develop haemorrhoids, which are caused by increased pressure on the rectal veins secondary to pregnancy. By straining to have a bowel movement, you put stress on the rectal veins, which can become blocked, trapping blood, turning itchy and painful, and perhaps even protruding from the anus. Exercise, a high-fibre diet and plenty of water can help to avoid constipation and straining with bowel movements that may aggravate the condition. Try easing the pain with an ice pack, a soak in a warm tub, wipes with witch hazel pads or a topical prescription cream as recommended by your doctor.

Haemorrhoids do have the potential to become more than just a minor discomfort, so be sure to speak to your doctor about them if they do occur. While they typically resolve after pregnancy, in some cases clotting occurs and surgery is necessary.

Other symptoms of second-trimester pregnancy you may start or continue to experience this month include:

· Nausea
· Fatigue
· Frequent urination
· Tender and/or swollen breasts

- Bleeding gums
- Excess mucus and saliva
- Increase in normal vaginal discharge
- Mild shortness of breath
- Lightheadedness or dizziness
- Wind and/or constipation
- Skin and hair changes
- Feeling warm or easily overheated

Movement!

Think that ultrasound was exciting? Just wait until you feel your little gymnast stretch and push inside you for the first time. If this is your second or third child, you may already recognize the familiar sensation of her little body flexing in your slightly used womb. For mums in their debut pregnancy with somewhat less stretchy accommodation, the first movements – known as quickening – may not be felt quite as early. By week 19, most women have felt that distinctive first flutter.

So what does it feel like? It's often described in terms of butterfly wings or bubbles, or less poetically as wind or a block of jiggling jelly in the abdomen. Because pregnancy can cause so many gastrointestinal symptoms, you may not even notice the gentle nudges of baby until she's been persistent with her movements for a few days.

You'll quickly discover that your baby is already establishing behavioural patterns. When you're up and about, she may be rocked to sleep by your movements. It's when you lie down and try to take a rest that she wants to get up and groove. Is your partner having a tough time getting a hand on your stomach in time to feel the foetal kung fu? Have him stand by during a down time and see if he can catch a kick or two.

Once baby starts moving regularly, the sensation quickly becomes second nature. On average, you should feel four or more movements each hour from your passenger. Three or fewer movements or a sudden decrease in foetal activity could be a sign of foetal distress, so if you notice either, call your doctor as soon as possible to follow up.

The Shape You're In

Carrying high or low? Looking large or barely showing? It's practically inevitable that at some point in your pregnancy someone will guess the gender of your child based on how he or she is filling out your belly. While guessing is a fun way to pass the time, the theory that high means a girl and low means a boy has no basis in science. How you carry depends on your build, posture and pregnancy history. Women who have had a previous pregnancy tend to have more pliable abdominal muscles and therefore often carry lower. The baby's position also influences your pregnant topography, which may change from one day to the next.

At the Doctor

If you didn't get a listen to the foetal heartbeat last month, you'll probably get your chance with this visit. Women who have chosen to take an alpha-foetoprotein (AFP) test will have their blood drawn sometime between weeks 16 and 18. For more on the AFP, see Chapter 5.

On Your Mind

You're now hitting your stride as the wooziness and uncertainties of the first three months fade away, and the discomforts of late pregnancy still lie relatively far ahead.

Feeling better and having more energy, you may be ready to conquer the world (or at least the nursery). Yet colleagues, friends and family, now starting to recognize you as 'a pregnant woman', may be handling you with kid gloves.

The pampering is nice, within limits. Accept the small favours that ease the discomforts of pregnancy – such as a closer parking space or the cushy chair in the conference room. But don't hesitate to be firm with those who try to pressure you to cut back on tasks you're perfectly capable of handling, or who treat you like a porcelain doll.

Reality Strikes

For many women, the starter's pistol on motherhood goes off when they feel baby's first pokes and prods. The palpable presence of your child may trigger a series of mothering emotions – protectiveness, nurturing, nesting – and complete and total impatience with anyone who poses a potential threat to the well-being of you and your child.

This maternal defense system may seem a bit extreme to the partner who is banished from the bedroom when he has a head cold, or the visiting friend who is asked to take his cigarette outside in sub-zero weather, but you aren't being paranoid or unreasonable. No one would think twice about keeping a newborn away from sneezing and smoking; a developing foetus is just as, if not more, vulnerable.

Are my vivid dreams related to pregnancy?
Dreams that are exceptionally realistic, disturbing or just plain bizarre are common in pregnancy. Your dreams are reflections of what's on your mind, so it's natural for them to reflect concerns about the baby, your family and the future. They may seem larger than life right now due to insecurities about the future and again, those pregnancy hormones.

Exercise

Don't avoid the gym, pool or other favourite fitness hangouts just because you're pregnant. Exercise will not only make you feel better, it can tone muscles that will be getting a workout in labour and delivery. Feeling alarmingly large among the gym babes? Try mixing up your routine with something new like walking, golf (no cart) or a prenatal exercise class.

So how much is too much? It depends upon your prepregnancy fitness level. If you were swimming one hour each day before pregnancy, there's no reason not to continue that routine if you have your provider's blessing. On the other hand, don't start training for a marathon if your notion of exercise is walking into McDonald's instead of taking the bus.

The rule of thumb – for women in 'regular' pregnancies (i.e. not high-risk), 30 minutes of moderate exercise daily is ideal.

Benefits

If you weren't into a regular fitness routine before pregnancy, exercise may be just about the least appealing thing you can imagine right now. Try to set your distaste aside for a few moments and consider the benefits a regular workout may provide: Do speak to your caregiver before beginning a new exercise routine.

- **Energy up.** Stretching and moving daily will boost your energy level and calm your mind.
- **Postpartum weight down.** It will be easier to work off your pregnancy weight after the birth if you already have a regular routine.
- **Ease your aches and pains.** Exercise that promotes strength and flexibility can prevent or diminish lower back pain, muscle aches and other complaints of pregnancy.
- **Positive mental attitude.** Feeling fit may improve your self-image.

Staying Active

Exercise doesn't have to be complicated, expensive, or technically difficult. It can be as simple as throwing a ball with the kids in the back garden, taking the dog on a brisk walk each evening, or swimming or even walking laps in the local pool. Again, 30 minutes of regular, heart-pumping activity, started and finished by a good stretching routine, is all it takes to benefit you and baby. Above all, make sure it's an activity you enjoy or something done in good company, so you will look forward to it.

If you thrive on routine and feel more likely to get moving if you have a set schedule, check out your local hospital or community centre for a prenatal exercise class. Water exercise programmes are also a good, low-impact way to get fit. Even if your class is tailored toward mums-to-be, check with your doctor first.

Certain activities are definitely off-limits during pregnancy. These include scuba-diving, water-skiing and contact sports. In addition, proceed with caution when participating in potentially high-impact activities like tennis, volleyball and aerobics. As always, run any new or pre-pregnancy fitness routine past your doctor before you take part.

Precautions

While exercise can be a boon to your body and baby, there are basic steps you should take to stay safe. First and foremost, check your routine with your doctor to get a medical stamp of approval. If you're new to working out, start slowly. Be attuned to your body's signals and stop immediately if you experience warning signs such as abdominal or chest pain, vaginal bleeding, dizziness, blurred vision, severe headache or excessive shortness of breath.

Dress in supportive, yet comfortable clothing that breathes well and braces your belly and other parts of your expanding anatomy. If your feet have swollen past the comfort level of your old gym shoes, invest in a bigger pair. Drink plenty of caffeine-free fluids before, during and after your workout to remain well hydrated, and try to work out in a climate-controlled environment to avoid an extreme rise in core body temperature, as overheating can be hazardous to a developing foetus.

Pelvic floor exercises are one exercise every pregnant woman should know and practice. They strengthen the pelvic muscles for delivery and can improve the urinary incontinence, or dribbling, some women experience in pregnancy. Tighten the muscles you use to shut off your urine flow, hold for four seconds, and relax. You've just done your first pelvic floor. Try to work up to ten minutes of exercises daily.

Just for Dads

Every couple bickers once in a while. In fact, many relationships seem to thrive on heated debate. But the hormonal tidal wave and stressors that accompany pregnancy may bring an unexpected degree of added friction to the mix. Try to remain sensitive to her physical and mental changes without being condescending or unsympathetic. In other words, 'Darling, I know it's just the hormones talking', is not a good way to resolve an argument.

Understanding Her Emotions

You can't feel her aches and pains, but you can feel the brunt of her volatile emotions.

Even if you understand why she's moody, with all this exposed emotional wiring, you may be tempted to keep a low profile. Remember, your partner needs empathy and assistance right now, not sympathy and avoidance. Support her with your actions, love and acceptance, and you can make it through this pregnancy with an even stronger bond.

You may be starting to feel the 'but what about me?' syndrome coming on. The hullabaloo surrounding your partner and your unborn child may be making you feel a little (or maybe even a lot) neglected. Your partner is focusing on the pregnancy and baby instead of you, as well. Feeling left out, or even jealous, is perfectly normal.

Try to address your feelings by arranging some special couple time for you and your partner where you both can be waited on and pampered a bit – splash out on a night out at a special restaurant, a weekend at a nice hotel or a double massage. And also keep in mind that you have a very special role to play in this pregnancy too – as father-to-be, both mum and baby are relying on your support, coaching, patience and love.

What You Can Do to Help

Be patient. You will be expected to use your mind-reading capabilities to their fullest extent. In other words, your partner may not ask for help, but you need to offer it (and offer it frequently). Then – and this is critical for the procrastinators among you – follow through soon after. If she is in nesting mode, chances are she won't let things sit undone for long. If you don't follow through, then all you've done is to compound her stress with irritation.

Volunteer for errands and chores that are starting to become physically difficult for her pregnant body, such as weekly trips to the laundromat, mowing the lawn and taking your ill-behaved St Bernard to the groomer. Let her sleep in at weekends. Take care of some of those household repair tasks you've been meaning to get to before she has to remind you about them.

If you already have other children, it's easy to let your partner's rest and mental health needs take a back seat as other parental responsibilities come to the forefront. Consider getting some extra help around the house from relatives or even a biweekly cleaning service to keep things manageable. Don't miss Chapter 11 for tips on helping your family adjust to second or later pregnancies.

Chapter 9

Working Through Pregnancy

Worried about keeping up on the job during your pregnancy? Recognize your value, not just as an employee but also as a woman. Don't let anyone make you feel guilty about being pregnant. Know your rights, stick to your guns and realize you don't have to settle for the status quo when it comes to the workplace.

Your Rights

Unfortunately, it's sometimes easier to change the legal employment landscape than alter prevalent workplace attitudes and prejudices. Remember that you are protected from discrimination by law (see Chapter 3). In addition, many employers pride themselves on offering generous conditions to working mothers (and fathers) to be.

Occupational Hazards

Depending on your position and work environment, you may have to alter your duties temporarily, or request a change in location or accommodation. If your job involves any of the following elements, talk to your personnel department about your options:

· **Weight-lifting.** Lifting heavy packages, boxes or other items is not recommended in pregnancy, especially past 20 weeks (e.g. shipping and receiving clerks, warehouse work).
· **Secondhand smoke.** Women who work in the hospitality industry (e.g. bartenders, waitresses) may expose their foetus to toxins in secondhand smoke.
· **High heat.** Excessive temperatures can be harmful to foetal development, particularly in the first trimester (e.g. summer construction, factory environment).
· **Chemical exposure.** Jobs that involve working with certain chemicals and hazardous substances (e.g. welders and lead exposure) are linked to birth defects.
· **Standing and repetitive movement.** Line work or other jobs that keep you on your feet all day (e.g. factory jobs, assembly work, piece-work) can exacerbate circulatory problems.
· **Ionizing radiation exposure.** Pregnant pilots and flight crew may be exposed to excessive ionizing radiation, another known teratogen. Radiographic imaging technicians who work with X-rays, CT scanning equipment, and nuclear medicine are also at risk.

Breaking the News

In an ideal world, the news of your impending motherhood would be greeted with congratulations and reassurance at the office. Instead, reality may find you fighting against a negative employer reaction and determining the right time to drop the pregnancy bombshell for minimal fallout to your career. That pregnancy should be considered a handicap to be overcome rather than the positive, life-affirming force it is remains a glaring reminder of how far women still have to go to achieve equality in the workplace.

When you do inform your employer, make sure that they hear it from you, and not around the water cooler, first. Accompany the news with your tentative schedule for maternity leave so your manager can plan accordingly. Offering suggestions you have for a replacement in your absence or ways to temporarily reassign workload will reflect well on you and your perceived commitment to your employer. For more on 'When (and What) to Tell Work', see Chapter 6.

Avoiding the 'Mummy Track' Trap

Once you share your news, you may suddenly find yourself on a slow road to nowhere at work – last in the information loop and out of the running for promotions and job advancements you were previously an easy pick for. Goodbye fast track and hello mummy track?

Is it unavoidable? Not necessarily. Employers who realize that a happy employee is more likely to be a productive employee won't punish you for pursuing a personal life. And if you continue to perform well and make it clear to your supervisors and management that you'd like to have a career path with the company rather than just a job, you're more likely to avoid the so-called mummy track. Still, whether the mummy track exists in your organization or not depends on the corporate culture and the attitudes of upper management. Do they support family-friendly policies? Do they lead by example and use benefits like paternity leave themselves? And are efforts made to institute initiatives that benefit employees across the board, from the security staff to the bosses?

The Ideal versus the Real

In the real world, some organizations 'reward' those who invest themselves more fully in the workplace than in family. The result is an atmosphere in which pregnancy is construed as a choice 'against' company and career, one that may be tolerated for the sake of political correctness but certainly isn't supported through policies and rewards systems. The good news is that there are family-friendly employers who put their benefits packages where their mouth is. Don't forget that you have rights, and your employer must respect these. You have a right to time off for all antenatal appointments, including classes. See where your company lies between these two extremes:

The ideal... a fully equipped lactation facility.
The real... a toilet cubicle with a broken lock.

The ideal... expectant mother parking spaces near the entrance.
The real... unless you have an acronym after your name, it's first come, first served.

The ideal... a pregnant supervisor to commiserate with.
The real... your boss is a freshly minted Business Studies graduate who thinks 'family-friendly policy' means Christmas off with pay.

The ideal... a flexible schedule for your unpredictable pregnant body.
The real... don't forget to sign out for toilet breaks.

The ideal... a fully supervised and funded crèche at your place of work.
The real... paying through the nose for out-of-hours childcare because your train was late.

Defining Personal and Professional Goals

What do you want out of life, both personally and professionally, now that your family is changing? If this is your first child, it can be hard to fully assess the new direction you're taking. But there are probably some basic decisions you can make with a degree of certainty. For example, late shifts and double-overtime may be out of the picture for you now.

You may also have career goals that you'd like to keep on target. Should they be mutually exclusive of motherhood? No. They may be, depending on where you work? Yes. If you wanted to move into a supervisory position at your next review, but see your company promoting those who work excessive overtime, you have choices to make. Such is the delicate balance of motherhood. Fortunately, you always have the option to look for a workplace that is more in harmony with your personal and professional goals – or to take your own path, whatever it may be.

Realize Your Value

Think of full-time motherhood as another job offer on the table for your employer to stack up to. Your company may be willing to sweeten the pot with flexitime, telecommuting or other family-friendly working arrangements to keep you happy. Remember, in most cases they have poured a significant amount of money and resources into your training. The loss of that investment, plus the cost of hiring and training a new employee, is a big financial incentive for keeping you on board. Don't be afraid to rock the boat. Realize your value and use it as a bargaining chip.

Negotiate Towards Your Goal

Think about using your maternity leave as a launch pad for alternate working arrangements. For example, if you would like more than the paid leave your company offers and would ultimately like some flexibility in your schedule, suggest a work arrangement like telecommuting for the six weeks following paid leave. By offering an alternative to your complete absence, you appear flexible and dedicated, and your employer certainly has nothing to lose by trying it. Even if you aren't prepared to take six weeks off unpaid should your employer turn you down, it's well worth the gamble to suggest the idea. You can always scale back your plans if your request isn't granted. And if it is accepted and works out well, you will have proven yourself for a more permanent arrangement down the road.

Practical Matters

No matter what your job, staying comfortable, relatively stress-free and economically secure during your pregnancy is essential.

Staying Comfortable

Women who work on their feet should make a habit of changing positions often and moving when possible. Wear comfortable shoes and consider support stockings.

For jobs that require a lot of sit-down time, make sure you have an ergonomically appropriate chair that promotes good posture. A lumbar support pad may also help ease pregnancy-related lower back pain, and you can put up your feet under your desk on a small stool or even a stack of phonebooks. If you are in a desk job, look for opportunities to get up and about. Take a walk to speak with a colleague instead of picking up the phone, or hand-deliver a memo instead of using inter-office mail.

Scheduling Doctor Visits

Hopefully, your employer recognizes that good prenatal care translates to a healthier, more productive employee and, in the long run, less time spent out of the office to care for sick kids. However, if you do face resistance in taking time off for doctor's visits, remember that prenatal care is considered necessary medical care and is a legal requirement. If all else fails, you can invoke your legal rights.

In the meantime, find out whether your doctor has evening, weekend or early-morning appointments that might fit around your workday. If you must go during office hours and your supervisor isn't pleased, offer her the alternative option of taking the entire day of your appointment off as holiday or unpaid leave instead. Perhaps she'll look at your short absence in a new light.

If you're getting flak for meeting basic prenatal care requirements now, just think what it will be like when you need time off to care for a sick child or keep another appointment. File a 'family-unfriendly' mental note for follow up post-pregnancy. Companies who score poorly in supporting their pregnant employees will probably continue the trend. If too many red flags are raised during your pregnancy, once you reach maternity leave it may be time to look for a company that realizes the value of both personal and professional fulfillment in their employees.

At the end of your rope with a real pain in the you-know-what? Write a no-holds-barred e-mail or letter to the person in question, but do not send it (leave his or her name off of it for now – there's nothing worse than hitting the send button by accident). Then let it sit overnight and revisit it the next day with a cooler and clearer head. Just airing your feelings will usually improve your outlook, and you can either edit it for tact and a PG rating, or send it straight to the shredder or delete folder.

Controlling Stress

The workplace can be a hotbed of stress. Deadlines, personality conflicts, difficult clients, quotas, overtime and more make for a pressure cooker that's not good for you or baby. Try to maintain some perspective and peace of mind by realizing that petty office politics mean little in comparison to the health and well-being of your child. Turn to Chapter 4 for tips on coping effectively with stress.

Maternity Leave

Your bonding time with baby should be free of workplace concerns. If you plan appropriately for your departure and absence as early as possible, you'll get more out of your time off. It's a good idea to put all maternity leave plans in writing for your supervisor and appropriate managers, and to make an extra copy to be placed in your personnel file.

Planning Ahead for Leave

Lay the groundwork for your maternity leave so there won't be too many questions or crises in your absence. If appropriate for your position, delegate some tasks to colleagues and arrange coverage by others. Find out if your supervisor plans on hiring temporary help to fill in during your absence, and work on training materials and checklists so you won't face a mess upon your return to the office.

Check and double-check that all appropriate benefits paperwork has been filled out, signed off and sent in well in advance of your planned departure. Maternity leave should be a low-stress time, not one that requires twice-weekly contact with the personnel department to find out the status of your disability claim.

How Many Weeks?

So just how much, or how little, maternity leave should you take? Certainly, the benefits your company provides will play a major factor in your decision. If you are in a position of some seniority, you may be able to swing an even longer leave by tapping into saved holiday time. Other factors to consider include:

- **Money.** How much time off can you afford if your maternity benefits are minimal or non-existent? Don't forget to add any money you'll be saving (i.e. dry-cleaning bills, lunches out, transport expenses) into your equation.
- **Management.** Even though you may be legally within your rights, in some organizations an extended maternity leave may be frowned upon by those above you. Consider what management might think, and more importantly, what kind of priority you should place on their disapproval.
- **Morale.** Are your colleagues and/or subordinates happy and motivated, or disillusioned and bitter? Employees who work as a team and feel appreciated in their workplace are more likely to rise to the challenge in your absence.
- **Malleability.** Does it have to be all or nothing? Think about offering some creative proposals for extending your leave, such as a reduced part-time schedule or telecommuting.

Evaluating your leave options will reveal the pluses and negatives in your company's attitudes toward personal employee fulfilment. If morale is poor and management is unyielding, once you've got past maternity leave it may be time to consider your options.

Back to Work

After you actually deliver your child, the toughest job you'll have is that first day back to work. You'll worry about whether his minder will be able to tell his hungry cry from his tired cry, if he's getting the attention he thrives on, and of course if he misses you. Try to focus on the benefits of the situation – the increased value of the time you do have together, his broadening horizons as he interacts with new children and adults, and the financial security your family is gaining.

Easing the Transition

No matter how you look at it, it's hard being away from your baby. If you can, go back on half days to ease into the separation. Drop in at day care during your lunch hour if it's logistically possible. Above all, make the most of the time you do have together by making home a work-free zone.

Striking a Balance

In your pre-mummy life, you may have set up certain expectations you find yourself hard pressed to live up to now. It's time to define appropriate work limits, even if it means pulling in old boundaries. Colleagues and clients who felt free to contact you before via pagers, mobile phones or what have you, day or night, now need to be gently guided to keeping it to the office, or at least evaluating the urgency of their issues before picking up the phone. Getting some control back may be as simple as gradually ridding yourself of all the extra gadgetry that makes you painfully accessible, and weaning your colleagues to voicemail or e-mail-only access.

Women who work non-traditional schedules may have special needs for achieving balance. Evening 'day care' can be hard to find without friends or relatives in the area, and scheduling that changes on a weekly basis can make child care even more difficult to plan on. Talk to your supervisor frankly about your needs, and see if a shift change or a more permanent schedule can be arranged. If you're a dependable and valued employee, your employer should rather work with you to retain your skills and experience.

Changing Paths

A corporate culture that was perfect for your single lifestyle may just not fit your new family way of living. If the nature of your job or employer makes it impossible for you to achieve that delicate work/home balance, it may be time to change direction with a new employer.

Family-Friendly Companies: What to Look For

Few organizations will admit to being family-*un*friendly when asked during the interview process. Uncovering the truth will take some detective work on your part.

Finding out about flexitime options when you're still in the interview process can be a sticky situation. In many organizations, arrangements like telecommuting are still reserved as a privilege or reward (or even a necessary evil) for those who have proven their value to the company. Unless the job description includes flexible arrangements, you're better off not inquiring directly about the possibility. Instead, ask broad questions about available benefits and the 'average' work day, which will reveal the information naturally.

You can look to resources like business-focused local and national media as a starting point. Corporate annual reports can also be a good source of information. Once your foot is in the door and you're going through the interview process, make sure you have an opportunity to talk to potential colleagues and get an overview of available benefits and programmes. A few programmes and plans that may be a good indication a company is family-friendly include:

- **Flexibility.** Does the company have written policies on options like flexitime, job-sharing and telecommuting?
- **Lactation facilities.** Are there appropriate, comfortable areas dedicated to breast-feeding or breast-milk pumping? If not, is your employer willing to provide an appropriate, private space?
- **Paid paternity leave.** Are dads given time off for a new baby with pay, or at least more than statutory? If a policy is in place, is it successful?
- **Onsite child care or child-care assistance.** Does your employer offer onsite facilities, or offer flexible working hours to allow you to pick your child up from the child minder on time?

Flexitime, Telecommuting and Other Options

Even if your company doesn't have established flexible working options, it can't hurt to put the idea to your supervisor or to the personnel department. There's always a first, and you may be blazing the trail for others who will follow you.

First of all, realize that your position needs to be conducive to the arrangement you're suggesting. If you have a computer-intensive desk job that could be performed remotely with a simple dial-up connection, you're more likely to get a telecommuting arrangement than a receptionist, whose job description requires her physical presence. Look at what type of flexible arrangement your position might mesh with. For example, job sharing might be perfect for the receptionist and a colleague.

Create a proposal that is well-researched and realistic. Outline just what you want from the arrangements, in specific terms including hours and logistical requirements (such as home computer equipment). Cover your contingencies, such as the ability to be available for onsite meetings, even if you aren't scheduled to be at the office.

Make sure you outline the potential benefits to your employer as well. For example, if office space is at a premium in your building, a tele-commuting arrangement will free your desk for other employees. If your employer has no track record of flexible scheduling programmes, the resulting boost in employee morale and company image is also a plus for their reputation.

I want to keep breast-feeding, but my company doesn't have lactation facilities. Any suggestions?

As more and more companies are seeing the value in family-friendly policies, perks like lactation lounges are becoming more commonplace. Talk to your personnel department about possible options at your workplace. Sometimes an unused storage area or empty office can be at least a temporary solution. If all else fails, you may be able to arrange something with a sympathetic colleague who has an office (with a door that locks so the copier repairman doesn't wander in). The toilet is the last resort, but it's exceedingly difficult to get milk to let down while you're balancing a pump and apparatus in a toilet cubicle. Also a pump can be *loud*, and the acoustics in toilets are good, which can add to the awkwardness.

Finally, the fact that you're making the suggestion reveals that you might consider greener pastures if your needs are not met. If that happens, your employer loses time, talent and money – the three things the corporate world wants to grow, not squander. Make it easy for them to say yes by putting together a well-considered and realistic proposal.

Full-Time at Home

Becoming a full-time mum is an exciting new venture for many women. If you can afford to stay at home without working for someone else, go for it. Pouring your skills and knowledge into parenthood can be enormously fulfilling, and is probably the most rewarding job you'll ever have.

Finally, for the woman who wants it all and wants it close to home, consider the possibility of forging your own family-friendly path. In today's wired world, many occupations lend themselves to home-based work – writing, income tax preparation, desktop publishing and Web design are naturals. If the field you currently work in is unfulfilling and you'd like to make a change, look at the hobbies you enjoy for some ideas – refinishing antiques, creating crafts for retail, sewing and painting are a few that might be a good fit for a new career. Starting something new is never easy, but sometimes just looking at the miracle of your child helps you to see the possibilities.

Chapter 10

Month 5

You're still enjoying the relative comfort level of the second trimester, but your energy and initiative may be slightly dampened by the dwindling quality of your sleep. Sleep deprivation can also contribute to mental fuzziness and emotional edginess. If you haven't done so already, start to value and prioritize time spent between the sheets (asleep, that is).

Baby This Month

At about 255–305mm (10–12in) long and somewhere around 454g (1lb) in weight, your baby has now reached the halfway stage of development in pregnancy.

▲ You and your baby at the halfway stage.

Your baby is starting to get a bit bulkier as she accumulates deposits of brown fat under her skin. This insulation will help regulate her body temperature in the outside world. She's using her bulk to make her presence known; if you weren't feeling her last month. you are likely to now. A look at her through ultrasound might reveal a wave of her clenched hands, which open and close freely now and have their own unique fingerprints.

The foetus is now covered in a white oily substance known as *vernix caseosa*, a sort of full-body foetal lip balm that keeps her fluid-soaked skin from peeling and protects against infection. Some of the vernix will remain on the baby at birth, particularly in the skin folds (more if she is early, less if she is post-term).

Your Body This Month

As baby grows, your muscles and ligaments stretch to support this new weight. The result may be a new set of aches and pains as your body adjusts to the load.

Your Body Changes

Feeling like you're being turned inside out? The skin of your belly (and accompanying button) is stretching, tightening and itching like mad. A good moisturizing cream can relieve the itching and keep your skin hydrated, although it won't prevent or eliminate *striae gravidarum*, or the dreaded stretch marks (no matter what the manufacturers claim for it). Whether or not you'll develop stretch marks is largely a matter of genetics, although factors such as excessive weight gain and multiple gestations may increase your odds of having them.

I was expecting stretch marks, but not varicose veins! What's going on here?
These hair-fine marks, also known as spider veins, usually appear on the lower legs and are caused when increased blood volume and pressure damage the valves that regulate blood flow up out of the blood vessels of the legs. The result is pooled blood in the vein and that telltale squiggly red or blue line. Wearing support stockings, putting up your feet, resting on your left side and taking an occasional walk when you need to stand for long periods of time can help to relieve leg soreness associated with varicose veins.

The red, purple or whitish lines of striae are created by the excess collagen your body produces in response to rapid stretching of the skin. They may appear on your abdomen, breasts or any other blossoming body part right now. Don't be too alarmed, as striae typically fade to virtually invisible silver lines after pregnancy. If you do feel self-conscious, there are some options for postpartum treatment of severe cases (see Chapter 21).

What You Feel Like

The band of ligaments supporting your uterus is carrying an increasingly heavy load. You may start to feel occasional discomfort in your lower abdomen, inner thighs and hips, called round ligament pain. Pelvic tilt exercises are useful for keeping pelvic muscles toned and relieving pain.

The pelvic tilt can be performed while standing against a wall, but may be most comfortable done kneeling on the floor. Keep your head aligned with your spine, pull in your abdomen, tighten your buttocks and tilt your pelvis forward. Your back will naturally arch up. Hold the position for three seconds, then relax. Remember to keep your back straight in this neutral position. Repeat the tilt three to five times, eventually working up to ten repetitions.

The root of all things uncomfortable – pregnancy hormones – also contributes to the lower back pain you may be experiencing. Progesterone and relaxin – the hormone responsible for softening your pelvic ligaments for delivery – are also loosening up your lower back ligaments and disks, and, combined with the weight of your growing belly, your back is feeling the strain. Women who are having twins or more are especially prone to lower back pain, which occurs in up to 50 per cent of all pregnant women.

If your abdominal and/or back pains are severe or accompanied by fever, vomiting, vaginal bleeding or leg numbness, call your doctor immediately. Most minor back pain during pregnancy is completely normal, but in severe cases it can also be a sign of preterm labour, kidney infection or other medical problems.

▲ Pelvic tilts can tone your perineum and ease pregnancy aches and pains.

A few tips to help you ease your aches and pains:

- **Stand tall.** Perfect posture can go a long way toward easing back pain. Try to keep your centre of gravity in your spine and pelvis rather than in your belly, which can give you a curved back.
- **Sit up straight.** Use good posture when you're sitting as well, and choose a chair with good lower back support. You can also purchase a special ergonomic support pad for your chair back, but a small pillow may do the trick just as easily.
- **Avoid twists and turns.** With everything so loose, a sudden move as simple as quickly turning at the waist to get out of bed may strain your back. Use your arms as support for a slow take-off when rising from a chair.
- **Practise your pickups.** If you have small children who still need to be lifted occasionally, it's essential to use good form. To avoid injury, bend and use your leg muscles to lift things, rather than bending from the waist and lifting with your back.
- **Warm up.** A warm pad on your back, hips or other sore spots may help relieve pain.
- **Sensible shoes.** Avoid high heels! They will place further stress on your spine, and they're anything but comfy these days.
- **Footrest.** Use a low stool or step to rest your feet when sitting. If you must stand for long periods, rest each foot on a step alternately.
- **Massage.** You now have a medical excuse to indulge in a regular back rub from your partner. A licensed massage therapist who is experienced in prenatal massage may also be helpful.
- **Fluff and stuff.** Sleep on your side with a pillow placed between your legs. This will align your spine and improve your sleeping posture. A full-sized body pillow or beanbag may help support your back and belly as well.
- **Exercise.** If you aren't doing them already, some stretching and flexibility exercises may be in order. Check with your doctor for approval and recommendations; if the pain is troublesome enough or if you have a history of back problems, she may suggest a physiotherapist to work with.

Feeling hot and bothered, and not in the fun sense? Pregnancy-induced changes in your metabolism and added weight may make you overheat. Dress comfortably, cool off in the shower or bath, and invest in a fan if you don't have air-conditioning.

Other symptoms you may start or continue to experience during this month include:

- Nausea
- Fatigue
- Frequent urination
- Tender and/or swollen breasts
- Bleeding gums
- Increase in normal vaginal discharge
- Excess mucus and saliva
- Mild shortness of breath
- Lightheadedness or dizziness
- Headaches
- Wind, heartburn and/or constipation
- Skin and hair changes

fact

If round ligament pain is an increasing problem, consider buying a belly support band or belt, available at many maternity and baby supply stores. These bands cradle your growing abdomen and may ease your ligament and lower back pain. Check with your doctor to see if one might be a good fit for you.

At the Doctor

If your doctor hasn't discussed counting foetal movements before, she may mention it now.

Now that you're halfway through pregnancy, you may be thinking more about labour and delivery issues. It's never too early to ask your doctor questions about what's on your mind. It's also a good time to start gathering information on childbirth classes from your local hospital or birth centre. There are several different methods of childbirth education, such as Lamaze, Bradley, and Bing; researching them now will give you and your partner time to learn more about which one is right for you. Even if you have experience in the delivery room, you can still benefit from a refresher course. Register early, but try to pick a class date that falls in your third trimester so the information will be fresh in your mind once the big day arrives.

Having a planned Caesarean? You'll still benefit from prepared childbirth classes, which typically offer a comprehensive look at the entire birth experience, including hospital policies and procedures, newborn care, and a sneak peek at the maternity ward and nursery. Mention your Caesarean when you call for information; some programs offer special classes just for moms who are having Caesareans.

On Your Mind

There's bound to be an uncomfortable episode or two while your emotions are so close to the surface. Couple this emotional tension with your ever-growing list of things to do, and tension is inevitable. Try to defuse the situation in time by having an action plan for coping with anger-provoking situations.

Irritability

Because of all the added demands on your body, mind and emotional balance, you may be finding yourself short on patience these days. In pregnancy, the proverbial molehill quickly becomes the mountain. You have absolutely no tolerance for the idiosyncrasies of others, and people you found mildly annoying before pregnancy may become absolutely impossible to be around.

If you can't stand your colleague's endless prattle about who did what to whom and got away with it, tell her you need some quiet time. And the next time your neighbour launches into her 303 easy steps for making your home look as great as hers, politely excuse yourself for a rest, rather than letting your boiling point rise. Pregnancy is the perfect excuse for steering clear of people who – let's face it – are just plain annoying. Of course, avoidance isn't the ultimate answer, but during this crucial time, when your emotional and physical balance are so important, it's a good solution for taking care of the little things and keeping your sanity intact.

If family and friends are getting your dander up as well, it may be a sign that you are feeling overwhelmed and undersupported. Take a look at what's really getting to you. When you blow up at your partner for forgetting to stop at the dry cleaners, is it because you really had to have your clothes back posthaste, or is it because you feel as though you have to either nag or do it yourself to accomplish anything? If it's the latter, sit down and tell your partner what you're feeling, and work out some strategies for easing the burden together.

Overwhelmed

Half your pregnancy has passed and gone, and the baby's room is a sea of boxes, you can't decide on a name, and your office isn't even close to being ready for your maternity leave. Step back and take stock. Are you making work and stress for yourself through self-imposed deadlines? Look at your 'to-do' list in terms of small tasks, rather than an all-or-nothing prospect. Prioritize what's there, and dare to cross off a few things that just aren't that important right now. It's nice to have everything *just so* for baby's arrival, but your new son or daughter is only going to care about three things – being warm, well-fed and near her mum and dad.

Also remember that you aren't in this alone. If you're single, enlist family or close friends to help out. And if you are in a couple but still aren't getting the help and support you need from your husband or family, ask for it. Although it's nice when others anticipate your needs and pitch in voluntarily, they may be wrapped up in their own preparations and anxieties about the new family addition. Don't feel guilty about reminding them that their help is needed now.

Sleeping Tight

Perhaps it's nature's way of preparing you for the sleepless nights to come, but your growing belly and the pushes and prods of your little one are making it increasingly difficult to get the requisite eight or more hours of peaceful slumber. Sleep is essential to your mental and physical fitness right now, not to mention that of your child. Make a big effort to rest often and rest well.

Making Time

You work a full day at the office, go to the supermarket, come home and make dinner, stay up late working on the baby's room, and next thing you know it's midnight. Sleep is a priority now, one you need to make time for. Make a regular bedtime, and stick to it. Leave major cleaning, errands and home projects for weekends or other days when you are off work or have extra help. If getting to bedy late is unavoidable, try to make up your sleep deficit with a weekend nap.

Getting Comfortable

The foetal sleep cycle is only 20–80 minutes long, so if you aren't a sound sleeper you may find yourself awakened by baby's stretching limbs. Getting comfy may be a challenge if you were a dedicated stomach or back sleeper before you were pregnant. Lying on your back puts undue pressure on your inferior vena cava, the vein that shuttles blood from your lower extremities (feet and legs) to your heart, and can trigger a drop in blood pressure. It's also extremely uncomfortable for any length of time at this stage. Both logistically and medically, the best position for sleep right now is on your side.

Left-side sleeping enhances blood flow exchange with the foetus. Why is the left side preferred? Because the liver resides on your right side, and sleeping on that side positions your heavy uterus right on top of it. That said, right-side sleeping won't really hurt anything in a typical pregnancy, so if you wake up on your right, don't panic.

Hip and shoulder pain may be another source of sleepless nights, and one that's difficult to avoid since you must sleep on your side. If you've tried the tips for aches and pains outlined above and the pain is still keeping you awake, experiment with a foam 'egg-carton' cushion on your mattress for a little added padding.

You don't know what living is until you've had the luxury of stretching out full (and pregnant) on an acre of crisp cool sheets. If you don't have one already, and it's affordable, think about upgrading to a king-size bed. The extra room enables you to bring a body pillow or bean-bag into bed to support your stomach and ease your back. Your partner will benefit, too, as he'll be less likely to wake at every toss and turn.

Another bedroom habit you may have picked up in pregnancy is snoring. Many women are mortified and self-conscious about this new development. After all, there's nothing that makes you feel more attractive than the thunderous vibration of your own nasal passages, unless it's waking up with a trail of dried dribble on your face! The snoring may be related to a number of factors, including pregnancy-related nasal congestion, your increased need for oxygen, swollen airway tissues, and compression of the muscles that control breathing. Most of the miracle remedies and devices advertised on TV or in newspapers and magazines will do little but cost you money. Your snoring will probably fade away after pregnancy, so for the moment, invest in extra earplugs for your mate instead.

If you have been experiencing regular, sleep-disturbing snoring, make a point of mentioning it to your doctor or midwife. In a 1999 study, Swedish researchers linked chronic snoring in pregnancy to high blood pressure, oedema (swelling), and low birth weight. They also found that habitual snorers were more likely to experience pre-eclampsia than infrequent or non-snorers. If you snored a lot pre-pregnancy, you could have a sleep disorder called sleep apnoea, which should be assessed by a doctor.

Make sure your environment is as sleep-friendly as possible. The room temperature should be cool enough for your overheated metabolism; your partner may want to stock up on extra blankets to get him through these occasional chilly nights. If ambient noise is a problem, get some earplugs or a white noise conditioner to cut the clamour. Keep a nightlight plugged into your room or hallway to navigate those inevitable late-night toilet breaks with minimal injuries.

More tips for preparing yourself for a good night's sleep:

- To avoid heartburn, don't eat immediately before settling down, and have an extra pillow on hand to elevate your head.
- Make the toilet the last stop before bed.
- Stock your bedside table with water biscuits if you still wake with an unsettled stomach.
- If tender breasts are keeping you awake, wear a jogging or other supportive bra to bed.
- Stay away from caffeine (it isn't the best thing for you at this stage anyway).
- Don't exercise within three hours of bedtime.

Just for Dads

Although your partner is still in the relative calm and comfort of the second trimester, you may be dog-tired, as her tossing, turning and expanding territorial stake of the bed have you sleeping fitfully. Some earplugs, or perhaps even an occasional night on the couch or spare room bed to recoup sleep losses, can be invaluable. You may also be thinking more, perhaps with some apprehension, about your impending dad duties. Instead of worrying, take action.

Practice Makes Perfect

It's often said that a new baby doesn't come with an owner's manual or instruction book, but that's not completely true. Most hospitals will offer you a small forest of literature on how to care for your child once you get him home. Between this, prenatal education classes and the hundreds of baby books at your local library and bookshop, you can at least gain an understanding of how all the parts are supposed to work.

However, if you're feeling a little insecure about your capabilities, getting some hands-on experience with a living, breathing baby can be a real plus. Offer to take care of a niece, nephew or neighbour's child so you and your partner can get some baby-care practice (Hint: don't use the word 'practice' when offering babysitting services to their parents). If you're not quite up to the flying solo skill level yet, the next time you're visiting take the opportunity to hold, feed or (if you're feeling daring) change the baby. Your interest will be welcomed; parents love an extra set of hands.

Some women experience restless leg syndrome, or RLS, in late pregnancy. Characterized by pain or unpleasant sensations in the legs that are only relieved by movement, the exact cause of RLS in pregnancy is not known. It may be related to nerve compression or an insufficient intake of folate and/or iron. If RLS is keeping you awake, talk to your doctor about treatment options.

The Second Time Around

Perhaps you're an expert at all this dad stuff already, and you've been coasting through this pregnancy with ease. You still have some unknowns to deal with, including how your existing child or children are going to handle the mantle of siblinghood. Don't forget that every pregnancy is different, and what could have been smooth sailing last time may be tougher this time around (or vice versa).

Also keep in mind that even though you don't have new dad anxieties to contend with, your partner still has to do the heavy work. Share child-care duties, take time to pamper her, and make her feel like a supermodel mum-to-be, rather than the old lady who lives in a shoe. For more on second or later pregnancies, see Chapter 11.

Chapter 11

Repeat Performance: Second or Subsequent Pregnancies

Maybe you've been through this before and consider yourself an expert at this pregnancy stuff. Even if the physical side of pregnancy is familiar, the emotional and mental aspects involved with each new child are always different. Families change with each new member – and yours will be no exception to the rule.

Baby and Your Body

Women who have been through pregnancy already (known as *multigravida* in clinical lingo) have some definite body benefits when it comes to carrying and delivering their baby. On average, labour is typically shorter, and these women are statistically less likely to need an episiotomy.

In addition, you'll probably feel your little one stirring earlier than your first, primarily because you can identify the sensation this time. Depending on the tone of your abdominal muscles, which may be laxer after your first pregnancy, you may also start to show earlier.

Every Pregnancy Is Different... Or the Same

In pregnancy, practice doesn't always make perfect. Just when you think you have it taped, Mother Nature may bowl you a bouncer. You may have been horribly nauseous throughout your first pregnancy, and not even have a wind bubble this time around. Or your second pregnancy may be filled with all sorts of strange, new symptoms. It's also possible that your second pregnancy may be a carbon copy of your first. Each baby has its own genetic blueprint, its own site of implantation and its own unique placenta. The environment and life circumstances each child is born into may be vastly different as well. On the other hand, all your pregnancies share the same maternal infrastructure, which may account for similarities in labour and delivery, pregnancy complications and so forth. So will this pregnancy be the same or different? You'll just have to wait and see.

VBAC or Another Caesarean?

'Once Caesarean, always Caesarean' is an out-of-date obstetrical concept. Although many factors are involved in the decision to repeat a Caesarean (e.g. high-risk pregnancy, foetal position, type of incision made in the first section, scarring of uterus, number of previous Caesareans), many women *can and do* try vaginal birth after caesarean (commonly known as VBAC). According to the BMA, the success rate of VBAC is between 60 and 80 per cent.

In the days before a transverse (or horizontal) Caesarean incision was the obstetrical norm, VBACs were often discouraged because of the risk of uterine rupture, which might occur when a weakened scar from a first Caesarean burst open under the pressure of strong contractions. Clinical studies have shown that prostaglandins can increase the chance of uterine rupture in VBAC, and the ACOG does not recommend their use in induced labour of VBAC for this reason. The use of oxytocin in a VBAC labor should also be closely monitored. (For more on induced labour, see Chapter 18.)

In women who are considered appropriate candidates for VBAC, vaginal delivery is often encouraged over Caesarean because of the potential complications involved with surgery (e.g. infection, haemorrhage). If you are having a VBAC, your doctor may advise you to be delivered in a hospital equipped to handle a Caesarean if one becomes necessary. The ACOG recommends this type of setting, but many midwives don't believe this is necessary in an uncomplicated pregnancy scheduled to deliver by VBAC. Again, this is highly dependent on your medical history. If you are considered to be at low risk, a home birth may be a reasonable choice for you. Talk to your doctor for her views on the situation.

Do keep in mind that another Caesarean will also require a longer recovery period than vaginal birth, something to consider when you already have children who must be cared for postpartum, in addition to your new baby duties. However, recovery may seem a bit faster than getting back on your feet after your first Caesarean, just because you've been through the process once and know what to expect.

Sharing the News

Don't be too disappointed if your news isn't met with the fanfare your first pregnancy announcement was greeted with. People tend to be a bit more laid-back in reacting to second or subsequent pregnancies, which actually may be a better approach in helping your children adjust to the news.

With an Only Child

Telling your other child or children may not be all you had imagined it would be, either. The reactions you get may run the gamut from happiness to horror. But involving the kids in the pregnancy from the beginning can benefit you all in the end. Even the child who has been begging for a little sister or brother will have some adjustments to deal with. If you know the gender of the new baby, it may have some bearing on how your child takes the news as well. Girls and boys who envisioned a resident same-sex playmate may be crestfallen when their plans change. Friends with siblings may give your child an earful on how boys and girls operate. Don't worry – your little one will eventually come around.

If you have a toddler or preschool child, consider waiting until the first trimester draws to a close to tell them . Your due date might as well be in ten years, considering how slowly time seems to pass from a young child's perspective. Adding this short delay may make the wait more bearable. Of course, there is no one-size-fits-all method – consider your child's unique temperament in deciding when to share the news.

Should you reveal the gender if you know it? You know your child, and her personality, best. For example, if she doesn't like surprises and takes a while to warm up to new situations, you may want to let her know so she can prepare herself (particularly if she's making grand plans for her sister, and a brother is coming).

If you have the opportunity, exposing your child to a friend or relative's baby may pique her interest in just how these little people work. Children who have absolutely no interest in sharing you may be coaxed into a more optimistic attitude if you're able to involve them in the pregnancy.

With an Older Sibling

Older children can be involved with your pregnancy much earlier, and will probably enjoy helping you consider new baby names, hearing the baby's heartbeat, seeing their sibling on the ultrasound screen and other milestone events of pregnancy. If they're old enough and have expressed an interest in helping out with baby care once their brother or sister arrives, you might even sign them up for a babysitting course through your local Red Cross.

In Stepfamilies

Blending families and stepsiblings can be a challenge at any age. Giving your children or stepchildren time to make a healthy adjustment to their new family unit prior to a pregnancy is probably the best way to set the stage for a new sibling. Even if your family is relatively young, all of you (especially stepsiblings) may be brought closer together by this new common bond in your family life.

Still, along with the uncertainties any child experiences about a new baby in the family, a stepsibling may question his place in the new family unit even more. Will the new baby replace him or her in your mind? Will she receive the lion's share of love and attention because both her parents live in the household? Involving the kids throughout the pregnancy, stressing their importance as siblings and being supportive when they struggle with the transition are the best ways to ensure your family comes through pregnancy stronger than ever.

On Your Child's Mind

Getting comfortable with the idea of having a sibling, sharing parents and potentially sharing a whole lot more will take a little time. Don't rush your child, or expect instant excitement at the idea of a new baby. Each kid adjusts in his own way, on his own schedule.

Keeping your child's life relatively consistent on other fronts can help him or her adapt to the new baby better. Now is probably not the time to start a potty-training push, a move to a new house or a change of day-care providers. Stay on an even keel so she doesn't get overloaded.

Of course, some transitions, such as starting school, may not be avoidable. If a change is to occur, make sure it is cast in a positive light and its significance is noted, even if your household is in pre-baby chaos. The first day of nursery school is a big deal, and should be treated as such.

Some household changes, like moving your child into a bigger bed so the new baby can have his crib, may seem small to you but may make your child uneasy and even resentful. If he has to move into a new room before baby's arrival, give him the chance to plan and decorate it. Even the youngest kids can have some input on the decorative scheme (e.g. Teletubbies or Peter Rabbit motif?).

Foetus Rivalry

Even before birth, your unborn child is taking a lot of your time and attention, especially in your other kids' eyes. Turning home life into a baby-centred universe, where every discussion involves their sibling's arrival, is a guaranteed way to get their guard up, and may even make them question their importance in the family. Of course, talking about the baby's arrival is inevitable and healthy, in moderation. Just make sure the discussions don't exclude your other children.

If pregnancy is making you experience symptoms like nausea and vomiting that have you running slower than usual, your child may blame his sibling-to-be for your condition: 'Mum can't go to the beach *again*. That baby is causing trouble already, and the little pipsqueak isn't even born yet!'

Assure your child that the way you are feeling is 'normal' and is not caused by their brother or sister directly, but is instead just a part of pregnancy. You might even relate stories of your pregnancy with him or her if it was also plagued by morning sickness or other discomforts.

What's Happening to Mum?

Younger children are generally clueless about how a baby comes into the world. Stories of baby-dropping birds and kids coming from under gooseberry bushes may have them thoroughly confused. A good age-appropriate children's book on the subject can help you communicate the mechanics of pregnancy and birth if you find yourself at a loss for words. There are a number of books available to help. A local librarian or health visitor should be able to point you in the right direction.

When talking about conception, pregnancy and birth with your child, there are a few things you need to remember:

- **Be straightforward.** Don't fall back on the stork. Age will make a difference in how much your child wants or needs to know, but when you do answer questions, try to call a penis a penis, not a willy, tinkler or other adorable euphemism (tempting though it may be). Giving your child the right words to explain what is happening to your body and his family is a way to empower him and demystify this sometimes scary process.
- **Minimize the minutiae.** At the same time, don't take them from fallopian tube through baby's head crowning. Not only will they be bored to tears, but they'll probably tune out shortly after the sperm meets the egg.
- **Answer all queries.** As pregnancy progresses and becomes more visible and therefore more real to your child, questions may start to form in his mind. How can the baby breathe? How will she come out? What's she doing in there? Open the door for communication, and ask your child occasionally if she is wondering about anything.
- **Make it relevant.** Kids love to hear stories about their own infancy and 'foetal life'. Pull out the baby book and home movies, and explain what life was like when they were the new arrival.
- **Explain the emotion.** Don't forget to let your child know why you've chosen to bring another family member into the fold. Let her be aware of the intense love surrounding the choice to conceive and to bring her a sibling she can love as well.

Once it becomes clear that a new baby is on the way, you may notice some behaviour regression in a young child. Wanting to use a bottle, having potty-training accidents and other 'baby' behaviour is her way of saying she still needs you. Don't get angry with your child for slipping back into old habits, but do reinforce positive behaviour and point out the pluses and privileges of acting like a 'big kid' (e.g. if you talk like a big kid instead of using baby talk, you can learn how to answer the telephone).

Needing Reassurance

Even the most well-adjusted, confident kid will need reassurance once in a while that he's still the apple of your eye. Don't let your world revolve around baby preparations so much that it overshadows special time spent with your other children. And make sure you give your child or children every opportunity to be involved with your family expansion so they can feel needed and wanted.

Involving the Sibling(s)-to-Be

Making your child a part of the pregnancy process is imperative to starting siblinghood off on a positive note. A kid who is relegated to the sidelines while everyone is focused first on your pregnancy and then on the baby is going to resent this new intruder, with good reason. Start the getting acquainted process before birth, and let your child talk and sing to her little sister or brother, help decorate the new baby's room and take on other important tasks.

Sibling Classes

Many hospitals offer classes for new siblings as a companion to their roster of childbirth education programmes. When done right, an 'official' preparation – complete with nursery tour, baby (doll) practice, and in some cases a diploma – can make even the most reluctant big brother or sister feel special and important in his or her new sibling's eyes.

Sibling classes can also give your child a chance to air his fears among peers and receive reassurance that he isn't alone in worrying about this squalling, needy creature that's moving in soon. Discussions about how other households are handling baby preparation, sleeping arrangements and mum's coming trip to the hospital can also address concerns that your child hasn't thought of or hasn't felt comfortable verbalizing.

Classes should be small enough for discussion and interaction with peers and the instructor, and should ideally be separated into appropriate age groups. See Chapter 14 for more on sibling classes.

fact

A good way to start the sibling relationship off on a positive note is to pick out a special gift from the new baby to his big brother or sister, and present it during their first meeting. Your new addition will be receiving copious amounts of attention, praise and gifts, so this little gesture may symbolize a lot to your other child.

Through the Ages

Preteens and adolescents might be more receptive to the idea of a new sibling, simply because they're entering a phase in their development where they are focusing less on you and more on friendships and their social circle. A 14- or 15-year-old doesn't 'need' you in the way a toddler, nursery-school or infant-school child does. You've already gone from 'mummy' to 'mum' in their eyes, and a baby doesn't pose the same threat for your affections.

The Second-Time Father

Dads often feel that they have a bigger role to play in a second or later pregnancy, as the lion's share of child care often falls to them while mum deals with pregnancy symptoms. This is a great opportunity for you to spend time doing things with your kids that your partner normally gets to handle, and to help them adjust to baby's upcoming arrival.

Of course, all this 'together time' can have its pitfalls, too. While you may find yourself appreciating your wife even more when you have to take on tasks that she seems to handle effortlessly on a daily basis, that awe may sour to resentment as you realize that things won't change back to the old way soon. If you feel overburdened, ignoring the problem is not the solution. Stress is bad for both of you, but particularly for the growing baby, who is the focus of these changes. Don't let it get the better of you.

Get help from nearby family members, or hire childminders and household help if necessary. Even a local senior-school student can be useful to your partner as a mother's helper. And remember that your older kids may be ready and willing to take on new responsibilities in the family. The key is to communicate how you're feeling without blame, and to work on a way to resolve the problem together.

Don't forget that your partner also has more to cope with this time around. It may be harder to find the time to offer some pampering when you have kids who need your attention, but be creative and try to do what you can to ease the burden. If she has primary responsibility for day-to-day child care, giving her a little time to herself – even if it's just enough for an evening walk or a 15-minute adult conversation with a close friend – is really essential.

Living Large: When You Choose a Big Family

One is wonderful, two is terrific, three – well, you're starting to lose me but I suppose I see the benefits. Four? Are you MAD? If you have chosen to have a big family, you are probably used to this kind of reaction. Or perhaps you're just getting into the sizeable stage now, and haven't learned to shrug off the 'when are you moving into the shoe?' comments yet.

Whether your reasons are religious, rooted in your own upbringing or simply spring from a desire to have a home bursting with life and love, the bottom line is – it's your choice and your family. Don't let others make you feel freakish or, worse still, that you're neglecting the children you already have, just because you choose to have more than the national average. A child is one of the greatest gifts you can give your family and the wider community.

The success of a family lies in parenting quality, not in offspring quantity (big or small). Ignore the nay-sayers and remember that there are pitfalls and positive sides to every family configuration. There are enough theories and studies on sibling personality traits and birth order psychology to fill a not-so-small library. Although they may be fascinating to read, trying to base your future family structure on them is next to impossible. Not every middle child will be the easy-going mediator of the family, and not every only child will be a hopeless perfectionist. Instead, use the lessons in them to avoid possible parenting pitfalls.

Chapter 12 ·

Month 6

By month 6, you may feel as though you'll be pregnant forever, but the final trimester will come and go before you know it. Take some time this month to enjoy your pregnancy, warts and all, and treat yourself to some of the indulgences that only a mother-to-be can pull off.

Baby This Month

Feeling a rhythmic lurch in your abdomen? Your little chap probably has the hiccups, a common phenomenon thought to be brought on by drinking and/or breathing amniotic fluid. They'll go away on their own, eventually; in the meantime, enjoy your little drummer boy and take advantage of the beat to let your partner feel the baby move.

▲ You and your baby at the six-month mark.

The once-transparent skin of your foetus is starting to thicken, and sweat glands are developing below the skin surface. He's over 305mm (12in) long now, and by the end of the month may weigh up to 0.9kg (2lb).

You hold more than your child within your uterus; you also are accommodating the origins of your grandchildren. If you're having a girl, your foetus has already developed an estimated 7,000,000 eggs in her ovaries by 24 weeks gestation. The eggs will be enveloped in small sacs called follicles as pregnancy continues, and by birth the number of eggs will have decreased to around 1,000,000.

Baby may now startle (or react) to a loud noise or other stimulation. Because his auditory system (the cochlea and pathways in the CNS) has developed enough to sense and even discriminate among sounds readily, he is becoming accustomed to your voice and others who talk 'to' him frequently. Studies have demonstrated that newborns show a clear preference for their mother's voice, and for songs they heard while in the womb. Now is a good time to brush up on your lullabies.

Some clinical studies have found an association between exposure to excessive noise during pregnancy and high-frequency hearing loss in newborns. And while you can wear earplugs, your baby doesn't have the luxury. To stay on the safe side, you may want to avoid concerts, clubs and other high-volume environments now. If your job involves heavy noise exposure, talk to your doctor about possible risks.

Your Body This Month

Your uterus extends well above your navel now. You may actually be seeing foetal movement across your abdomen as baby gets comfortable in his shrinking living space. As baby seems to get more nimble, you feel exceedingly clumsy – breaking everything that isn't nailed down, tripping over your own swollen feet and taking out low-lying knick-knacks with your burgeoning belly. Blame it on your shifting centre of gravity, and be careful if you're walking in slippery or icy conditions.

Your Body Changes

If the shoe fits... consider yourself lucky. Few women are able to fit into all their usual shoes for nine whole months. What's behind all the swelling?

The dramatic increase in blood volume you've experienced in order to nurture your child is feeding excess fluids to surrounding tissues, resulting in oedema (or water retention). To make matters worse, the weight of your uterus is requiring the veins in your legs to work twice as hard to pump all that extra blood back to the heart. And, of course, another culprit is (say it together, everyone) – pregnancy hormones, as oestrogen increases the amount of fluid your tissues absorb.

The result of all this is puffy and sometimes aching feet. Putting your feet up when you can, wearing comfortable low-heeled shoes and soaking your feet in cool water are all good ways to ease the discomfort. Special support stockings, available at pharmacists, may also be helpful.

Don't restrict fluids or sodium – although avoiding excess sodium intake is fine, you actually need slightly more sodium in your diet in pregnancy to maintain your electrolyte balance. Fluids are also crucial to prevent dehydration and keep you and baby well.

If you experience sudden and severe swelling of the face and hands, call your doctor immediately. It may be a sign of pre-eclampsia, or toxaemia, a condition that is potentially hazardous to both you and your baby. Other signs of pre-eclampsia include high blood pressure, headaches, visual disturbances, sudden excessive weight gain and protein in the urine. To learn more about pre-eclampsia, see Chapter 13.

What You Feel Like

You may have added leg cramp to your list of pregnancy complaints. Stretching out your calf muscles can often get rid of cramp, so the next time it starts, extend your legs and point your toes toward your head. Some doctors suggest calcium supplements to ease cramp, but clinical studies are inconclusive as to whether or not this treatment is effective (although it can't hurt, given your increased calcium needs). A number of studies have found that oral magnesium supplements can be useful in alleviating cramp in some women. See what your doctor suggests.

Leg cramp can also be triggered by compression of your sciatic nerve –

a condition commonly known as sciatica, which can also cause numbness and burning pain down the length of your leg and in your lower back and buttocks. Try stretching, a warm compress or a soak in the bath for relief. And if you haven't already, review the tips for dealing with lower back pain in Chapter 10. If sciatica becomes more than a minor annoyance, talk to your doctor. A date with a physiotherapist may be in order.

If your leg pain is accompanied by swelling, redness and skin that is warm to the touch, call your doctor to report your symptoms. You may be experiencing deep vein thrombosis (DVT), a blood clot in your leg that impedes circulation and has the potential to embolize, or break off and block a major blood vessel. Pregnant women are five times more likely to develop DVT than their non-pregnant peers, due to a slow-down of blood flow and an increase in clotting factors. However, DVT itself is relatively rare, occurring in less than 1 of every 1,000 pregnancies. If DVT is diagnosed, intravenous anticoagulant drugs are typically prescribed to treat the clot, and bed rest may be advised.

Can the seat belt in my car hurt the baby? Should I stop wearing a shoulder belt?
Definitely continue to wear a seat belt throughout your pregnancy. The lap belt should fit snugly under your belly bulge, and the shoulder belt should be positioned between your breasts. Don't worry about the belt hurting the baby; the uterus and fluid-filled amniotic sac are excellent shock absorbers. It's much more dangerous to you and your child to go beltless and risk being thrown from the car or into the dashboard in an accident. You can also buy a clip-on attachment to make yourself comfortable.

Other symptoms on the menu yet again this month include:

- Nausea
- Fatigue
- Frequent urination
- Tender and/or swollen breasts
- Bleeding gums
- Excess mucus and saliva

- Increase in normal vaginal discharge
- Mild shortness of breath
- Lightheadedness or dizziness
- Headaches
- Forgetfulness
- Wind, heartburn and/or constipation
- Skin and hair changes
- Round ligament pain or soreness
- Lower back aches
- Mild swelling of legs, feet and hands

On Your Mind

Now that your belly is too big to *not* notice, it becomes somewhat of a conversation piece. At first, you may be surprised to find women you don't know asking about your due date or the gender of your baby. The next question will inevitably be 'Is this your first?' Welcome to the sisterhood of motherhood.

The 'What If' Game

Every new mum-to-be spends some time worrying about the health of her unborn child, especially if she's in a high-risk pregnancy. Take comfort in the fact that you've almost made it to the third trimester and your chances of delivering a healthy and happy baby are increasing each and every day. Obsessing over what could go wrong, rather than focusing on living well, will accomplish nothing but stress, insomnia and anxiety – three things that are bad for you and baby. If you haven't already, turn to Chapter 4 for more information on stress management, and read on for some stress-busting techniques to release your worries and relieve your mind.

Enjoying Your Pregnancy

As you come up to the third trimeste, try to take advantage of these final days of relative comfort and enjoy – yes, *enjoy* – your pregnancy.

Pamper Yourself

Splach out on a day spa treatment. Spend a lazy afternoon curled up with a good book. Cool off with a dish of your favourite ice-cream while you enjoy a nice relaxing soak in the bath. Take a pleasant weekend drive with no deadlines or particular destination. Pampering yourself can relieve pregnancy symptoms, give you (alone or with your partner) special time to reflect on your future, and recharge you for what lies ahead.

Make sure you treat yourself to the little conveniences right now, too. Use the park-and-ride service instead of walking from the car park, or shop where there is expectant mother parking near the shop's entrance and exit. Too tired to cook at the end of the day? Order a healthy takeaway from your favourite restaurant. If it's only lunchtime and you're already worn out, arrange for the kids to play at someone else's home for a few hours, and have a mid-afternoon snooze. It may feel decadent at first, but taking the easy way out is a good thing right now.

Don't Get Stressed

It bears repeating – again – that becoming stressed these days just isn't worth it for you or your growing child. Of course, pampering yourself is a good way to lighten the load. But some women find they just can't enjoy an old-fashioned self-indulgence day because they're too busy worrying about all the things they should be doing instead. If you fall into this category, don't add to your burden through forced relaxation that will only leave you tense and perhaps a lot poorer to boot.

Instead, use that money to whittle down your 'to-do' list. Use a cleaning service, send out the dry-cleaning, pay someone to do that painting in the baby's room, get the shopping delivered instead of trundling to the supermarket. If your financial resources are limited, let your loved ones know you could really use their help right now, and don't be shy about delegating tasks when assistance is offered

Spending Time with Siblings-to-Be

Watching your child marvel at the changes in your body while he considers the possibilities of a new little sister or brother can be one of the most fun and fulfilling parts of pregnancy. Yet even the most enthusiastic sibling-to-be has some doubts about how he will fit into the new family unit. Unfortunately, those insecurities may only be intensified as you spend more time in the coming months visiting the doctor, going to childbirth classes and tying down loose ends before the big day. Make sure you and your child or children have an opportunity each day to play, read or just talk. You'll both benefit from this special time together.

Couple Time

With you in the pregnancy limelight and all the attention your agile, rib-thumping foetus demands, you may have inadvertently started to think of you and the baby as a couple. Your husband or partner is not an orbiting moon, although he may feel like one from time to time. Make sure he knows that he plays a valuable role in this pregnancy, and take the time to reconnect with him emotionally and physically.

If these are your final few months as a childless couple, take advantage of your freedom and spend some time doing your favourite grown-up things, activities that don't involve visiting the doctor's office or shopping for cots and buggies.

If you're both still ready, willing and up to the challenge, sex can be more fun than ever. You don't have to worry about birth control, and the creativity required to find a comfortable position may inspire you to new heights. If the two of you are so inclined, oral sex may be a good option; just make sure your partner is aware that he should not blow into your vagina due to the rare but real risk of an air embolism. Women in high-risk pregnancies should consult their doctor about the safety of intercourse at this stage.

Just for Dads

Pregnancy is a special, one-of-a-kind time in your life, as well as your partner's. From 'My boy can swim!' to 'Breathe, darling, breathe!', this long, strange trip brings elation, anxiety, anticipation and much more.

It will also give you the opportunity to see your partner in a whole new light: to watch her grow physically and personally as she makes the amazing transformation to motherhood. Her strength and sheer stamina in this nine-month marathon may make you feel proud and protective.

A Brand New Lifestyle

Yes, life will change significantly once your child arrives. No running out to catch a late film and dinner at your favourite restaurant. You've got Disney matinees and Happy Meals on your dance card. Tinky-Winky and his smiling companions will eventually push your Monty Python video collection off the shelf . But the first time your daughter smiles at you, or says your name or laughs out loud at jokes that no one else would, it will all be so very worth it. And before you know it, you'll actually start to enjoy this second edition of your childhood from the parent perspective.

f@ct

Planning on taking her out for a nice romantic dinner? Some advance planning will make the evening more enjoyable. If you can, pick a restaurant that is completely smoke-free; even designated non-smoking areas can smell of lingering cigarette smoke if ventilation is poor. Make reservations so she won't be waiting on her feet for too long, and ask for space to give her more room to spread out. With her sometimes-fickle stomach, now is probably not the time to get adventurous with new cuisines, so stick to something tried and true.

Dads Should Enjoy Pregnancy Too

Unfortunately, even though we're well past the pacing waiting-room dads of the 1950s, fathers often get shut out of the pregnancy experience. The result can be frustration and anxiety. Many fathers-to-be experience significant stress related to the upcoming pressures of parenthood, but everyone's focus on mum and baby can minimize your concerns and leave you feeling excluded.

It isn't just a matter of the 'What about me?' syndrome. Dads who do try to connect with the pregnancy on a deeper level are sometimes ridiculed for their efforts. Ever get laughed at when you tell others 'We're pregnant'? Or perhaps you're the type who sniggers when the other guy announces his pregnancy (come on, you know who you are). Either way, you may end up internalizing your questions and fears due to a misguided sense of stoicism and consequently distancing yourself from the pregnancy experience.

Obviously, you'll never be able to fully experience pregnancy in a physical sense (nor will you probably want to, after watching the woman you love live through it), but you can increase your emotional investment in this pregnancy by communicating with your spouse or partner about your hopes, dreams and anxieties. Feeling stressed about your ability to be a good parent, or about how your relationship with your partner may change, or about the possible coming financial changes in your family, is completely normal. Talking about these issues as a couple can bring you closer together and help alleviate your worries. And the next time someone scoffs at 'your' pregnancy, you might remind him that without you boys, there would be no baby.

Chapter 13

Special Concerns in Pregnancy

Health problems, both those that pre-date your pregnancy and worrying symptoms and conditions that pop up during the gestation, can be difficult to deal with. Staying educated and informed can reduce related stress and will help you take the best care of both baby and your body.

Chronic Illness and High-Risk Pregnancies

If you have a chronic illness, such as type 1 diabetes, you'll probably be referred to a consultant early in pregnancy. Open communication during this critical time is absolutely essential; if any of your providers aren't willing to be team players, find someone who is.

You will be making more frequent visits to all your health-care providers throughout pregnancy to ensure that your illness remains well controlled and is not adversely affecting your unborn child. Any conditions that may potentially be transmitted to your child (e.g. HIV, herpes) either in the womb or during delivery may require drug therapy and/or potential Caesarean section as well.

If you have concerns about your child inheriting your condition, a trip to a genetic counsellor can be extremely helpful.

Your baby's development is mapped by the 46 chromosomes inherited from his or her parents (23 from mum and 23 from dad). Genetic blood testing of the parents can reveal if they are 'carriers' of certain hereditary conditions that may be passed on to their child. Testing of foetal DNA through amniocentesis or CVS can diagnosis a chromosomal abnormality while the foetus is still in the uterus.

Genetic Testing/Counselling

Couples who are considered at risk for certain pregnancy problems due to age, ethnicity, family history or a history of repeated miscarriage may be referred to a genetic counsellor for a risk assessment. You may be given the option for further genetic testing – which may include alpha-foetoprotein (AFP), amniocentesis, chorionic villus sampling (CVS) or ultrasound – and provided with detailed information on the conditions in question.

Hereditary and chromosomal conditions that genetic testing can reveal include, but are not limited to:

- Downs syndrome
- Trisomies (three copies of a chromosome instead of two)
- Tay-Sachs disease
- Sickle-cell anaemia
- Cystic fibrosis

Genetic testing can also reveal certain birth defects. For more details on what to expect from a visit with a genetic counsellor, see Chapter 1.

Ectopic Pregnancy

Ectopic pregnancy occurs when implantation takes place outside the endometrial lining. In the majority of cases, it occurs in the fallopian tube, which is why it is often referred to as a tubal pregnancy. However, an ectopic pregnancy may rarely also implant itself in the ovary, cervix, abdominal cavity or cornual portion of the uterus (close to the fallopian tubes).

Unfortunately, pregnancy implantation must occur in the endometrium of the uterus for a pregnancy to safely continue. Allowing a pregnancy to progress in the fallopian tube or other ectopic site will result in tubal or other rupture in the first trimester, unavoidable foetal death and potential maternal death. If you are diagnosed as having an ectopic pregnancy, it will need to be surgically removed or treated with the drug methotrexate. Early treatment can preserve your fertility for subsequent pregnancies.

Women who have had previous ectopic pregnancies, who become pregnant with an IUD contraceptive device in place, who have a history of endometriosis and/or pelvic inflammatory disease (PID) and who have had a tubal ligation procedure are at a higher risk for ectopic pregnancy. Approximately one in 100 pregnancies is ectopic.

Early signs of ectopic pregnancy include low hCG levels (hCG should approximately double every two days in a normal pregnancy), irregular bleeding, and pain. An abdominal or transvaginal ultrasound can usually confirm the diagnosis. If it remains undiagnosed, ectopic pregnancy is potentially life-threatening and can endanger future fertility. Warning signs that an undetected ectopic pregnancy may have ruptured include:

· Severe abdominal and/or pelvic pain
· Vaginal bleeding
· Dizziness
· Shoulder pain
· Nausea and vomiting

If you experience any of these symptoms, seek medical care immediately.

Our ultrasound detected choroid plexus cysts in our baby's brain – what does that mean?
If no other abnormalities were seen on the scan, these small cysts that appear on the choroid of the brain have an excellent chance of resolving themselves by around 24 weeks with no ill-effects to your child. The cysts are of note because in a small number of cases they have been associated with the serious chromosomal abnormality trisomy 18 (Edwards syndrome). Ultrasound technology has become so advanced in recent years that it is able to pick up more anomalies like choroid plexus cysts earlier and earlier, anomalies that statistically tend to mean nothing in most low-risk pregnancies. A meeting with a genetic counsellor will help you weigh the risks and benefits of further testing in your particular situation.

Molar Pregnancy

Like an ectopic pregnancy, a molar pregnancy is also not viable. However, in a molar pregnancy, the implantation site is normal but the embryo is not. Called a hydatidiform mole, this placental tissue develops into a mass of cysts that are often described as resembling a cluster of grapes. There are two types of molar pregnancy, complete and incomplete (or partial).

A complete molar pregnancy occurs when an egg with no genetic material inside is fertilized by one or two sperm. Most have 46 chromosomes, all from the father (paternal). The pregnancy itself contains placental mass only, and no embryonic tissue.

A partial molar pregnancy will usually contain some embryonic or foetal tissue. The majority of partial molar cases have two sets of paternal chromosomes and a single set of maternal chromosomes (69 in total).

Symptoms of molar pregnancy include:

· Too small or too large uterus for date
· Enlarged ovaries
· High hCG levels
· Vaginal bleeding
· Pre-eclampsia and toxaemia (if diagnosis is delayed)

Ultrasound can make a definite diagnosis of molar pregnancy. Older women have a higher risk for the condition, and the risk of subsequent molar pregnancy increases with each occurrence.

Removal by dilation and curettage (D & C) is the typical treatment for molar pregnancy. D & C is a surgical procedure involving dilating the cervix and suctioning the contents of the uterus. Synthetic hormones (oxytocin) may also be administered during the procedure to induce uterine contractions.

A molar pregnancy has the potential to develop into a rare type of cancer known as choriocarcinoma. Once the D & C procedure is complete, the uterine materials are examined by a trained pathologist to ensure that they are not malignant.

Gestational Diabetes

Gestational diabetes mellitus, or diabetes of pregnancy, is caused by a problem processing the glucose (or blood sugar) in your bloodstream. Glucose is important to the body, providing fuel for cellular growth and metabolism. To be processed effectively, glucose requires a companion hormone known as insulin. Insulin facilitates the transfer of glucose into the cells where it is metabolized, or processed for energy. With not enough insulin, or insulin that the body isn't using effectively, the result is a backing up of glucose into the bloodstream, a situation that is potentially damaging to all your organ systems and a developing foetus.

When you develop gestational diabetes, your pancreas is still making plenty of insulin, but your body isn't processing it efficiently. The condition, known as insulin resistance, is caused by certain placental hormones that counteract the effect of insulin (e.g. oestrogen, cortisol and human placental lactogen, or HPL). In most women, the condition doesn't reach critical levels, and their blood sugar levels stay within normal ranges. In others, excess blood glucose accumulates to potentially dangerous levels and treatment is required.

The Odds

Factors that may make you more likely to develop GDM include obesity, a family history of diabetes, a diagnosis of GDM or large birth weight babies in previous pregnancies and being over the age of 25.

Diagnosis and Treatment

Because blood-sugar levels are influenced by dietary intake, your doctor will probably try to treat your GDM with lifestyle and nutritional changes at the onset. A visit with a certified diabetes educator (CDE) and a registered dietitian (RD) can be invaluable in learning more about healthy menu planning, exercise and the basics of blood-sugar control.

You will have to self-test your blood glucose levels on a regular basis with a home meter. The home meter uses a lancet to prick your finger, arm or another test site for a blood sample. The blood droplet is placed on a test reagent strip that goes into the meter, and the meter provides a blood glucose reading. Testing is generally recommended first thing in the morning (a fasting test), and after meals (postprandial) – usually at one hour and again at two hours after eating. Your doctor may recommend testing at additional times, such as after exercise, if he feels it is warranted. Refer to the table overleaf to see what blood glucose levels the American Diabetes Association recommends for women with gestational diabetes.

If you don't experience significant improvement with dietary changes and your glucose levels still exceed normal ranges, you may have to take insulin injections to keep your blood sugar under control. Injections are typically taken before meals, to counteract their impact on glucose levels. Insulin does not cross the placenta and is not harmful to the development of the foetus..

Possible Long-Term Health Effects

Without proper treatment, uncontrolled blood glucose levels can result in foetal death or a condition known as foetal macrosomia (a baby that is too large). Blood glucose crosses the placenta in high levels, and the foetus responds by producing more insulin to process the load. The extra glucose is ultimately stored as fat, and the baby potentially grows too large for vaginal birth.

Women who develop gestational diabetes have an increased risk of a diagnosis of type 2 diabetes later in life, and should receive regular screening for the disease. Their children are also at risk for both type 2 diabetes and obesity. Fortunately, clinical studies have also shown that lifestyle changes involving regular exercise and a healthy diet can be extremely effective in preventing the onset of type 2 diabetes.

Newborns of GDM mums may also suffer from hypoglycaemia (or low blood sugar) at birth as they are suddenly 'disconnected' from the maternal surge of glucose and their high insulin production causes their blood-glucose levels to plummet. They may also have an imbalance of blood calcium and blood magnesium levels at birth. Because of these risks, a neonatologist may be on the scene during labour and delivery to treat any potential complications.

Hyperemesis Gravidarum

Hyperemesis gravidarum is excessive nausea and vomiting of pregnancy (i.e. morning sickness) that goes beyond the normal gastrointestinal disturbance experienced by many women. Its exact cause is unknown. The condition is diagnosed when nausea and vomiting trigger one or more of the following symptoms:

- Weight loss of 4.5kg (1lb) or more
- Ketosis
- Dehydration
- Electrolyte imbalance

Other conditions that can cause similar symptoms – including hyperthyroidism, pancreatitis, gall bladder or liver disease, gastritis, appendicitis and ectopic pregnancy – should be ruled out before diagnosing *hyperemesis gravidarum*. Treatment typically involves intravenous therapy to rehydrate and encourage weight gain (parenteral nutrition). Hospitalization may be required, and medications may also be prescribed.

Fortunately, *hyperemesis gravidarum* is relatively uncommon. For more on nausea and vomiting in pregnancy, see Chapter 2.

Incompetent Cervix

An incompetent cervix is a cervix that starts to open (efface and/or dilate) prematurely. It may be caused by a multiple pregnancy (twins or more), genetic factors, prior surgeries or a history of abortion. If your mother took the drug DES (diethylstilbestrol) when she was pregnant with you, you may also be at risk for an incompetent cervix.

As pregnancy progresses and your unborn child grows and places more pressure on the cervix, an incompetent cervix may result in miscarriage without treatment. Women who have had problems with incompetent cervix in previous pregnancies, or are considered at risk due to multiples, may be regularly monitored using transvaginal ultrasound to detect any cervical changes. If you ever experience vaginal bleeding or blood-tinged discharge, let your doctor know immediately.

Surgery to suture (stitch) the cervix closed, called a cerclage, may be recommended to prevent premature cervical opening. There are several different methods of cerclage, including the Shirodkar, the McDonald and abdominal cerclage. The most common type, the McDonald, is a temporary suture that is removed when labour begins. Another treatment option may be an appliance called a pessary, which is inserted into your vagina to support your cervix and uterus. Finally, bed rest may be prescribed to keep weight off your uterus, and abstinence from sexual intercourse will probably be recommended.

DES daughters, or women who were exposed to the drug DES (diethylstilbestrol) while in their mother's womb, are at risk for an array of health problems. If your mother was treated with DES (which she may be familiar with as synthetic oestrogen) between 1940 and 1971, particularly in the first five months of pregnancy, the drug may have affected the development of your reproductive organs. DES daughters are at a higher risk for miscarriage, preterm birth, ectopic pregnancy and a rare form of cancer called clear cell adenocarcinoma.

Intrauterine Growth Restriction (IUGR)

Intrauterine growth restriction (IUGR) occurs when foetal weight and size gain are estimated to be below the tenth percentile for gestational age. Some IUGR babies may be preterm, but others go to full term. IUGR occurs in up to 10 per cent of pregnancies.

Possible causes of IUGR include the following:

· **Multiple gestations.** IUGR occurs in at least one foetus in up to 20 per cent of twins or higher multiple pregnancies.
· **Infection.** Infectious agents such as toxoplasmosis and cytomegalovirus.
· **Placental problems.** Placenta previa, accreta or abruption, along with other placental abnormalities.
· **Umbilical cord compression.** Knots or twisting may decrease foetal blood supply.
· **Maternal hypertension.** High blood pressure in pregnancy, including pre-eclampsia.
· **Maternal tobacco, alcohol and drug use.** Smoking mums-to-be are almost twice as likely as non-smokers to have a low-birth weight baby.

- **Poor maternal nutrition.** Malnutrition and inadequate protein intake can restrict foetal growth and may lead to adult health problems, such as hypertension and insulin resistance, later in life.
- **Genetic anomalies.** Arrested physical and mental growth are two of the features of many chromosomal disorders, including Downs syndrome and Edwards syndrome (Trisomy 21 and Trisomy 18).
- **Birth defect.** Birth defects, such as a congenital heart or kidney malformation, may restrict blood flow and affect foetal growth.
- **Altitude.** The reduced oxygen supply at high elevations decreases blood flow to the uterus and placenta, and is thought to be a factor in IUGR and low birth weight.
- **Certain chronic illnesses.** Maternal heart disease, sickle cell disease, diabetes and systemic lupus erythematosis (SLE, or lupus), among others.

A fundal height (uterus height) that is measured as too small for the due date is the first tip-off to IUGR. An ultrasound can give your provider an idea of actual foetal size, and if IUGR is diagnosed you will probably undergo regular ultrasounds, non-stress tests and biophysical profiles through the remainder of pregnancy to follow your baby's progress (see Chapter 5 for more information on these procedures).

IUGR pregnancies are at risk for intrapartum asphyxia (blocked oxygen flow to foetus), oligohydramnios (low amniotic fluid volume) and possible preterm birth and its related complications. At birth, IUGR babies are at risk for a number of medical problems, including high blood pressure, hypoglycaemia (low blood sugar), anaemia, polycythemia (an excess of red blood cells), neurological problems and jaundice. Later in life they may experience some developmental problems.

What's the difference between IUGR and a preterm baby?
Preterm babies are typically also low birth weight (LBW), but they are still considered the appropriate size for their actual gestational age (time spent in the womb). Newborns diagnosed with intrauterine growth restriction, on the other hand, may be born at full term and *still* be small for gestational age (SGA). So in an acronym nutshell, non-IUGR preterm babies are LBW but not SGA, while IUGR babies (who can be preterm or full-term) are both LBWand SGA.

IUGR that begins early in pregnancy and affects the foetal body uniformly is said to be symmetric. Symmetric IUGR may be caused by genetic abnormality, foetal infection or exposure to teratogen. Growth restriction that occurs later in pregnancy and is thought to be caused by insufficient foetal nutrition is termed asymmetric IUGR. It is also called head sparing IUGR because the foetus has focused its limited resources on vital brain development, making the head in these babies much larger than the body. Asymmetric IUGR infants typically have a better prognosis, or long-term outlook.

Placenta Problems

The placenta provides nourishment, blood and oxygen to your baby, and is literally what connects the two of you. Problems can occur with either the structure or the placement of the placenta, which may pose a risk to you and your unborn child.

Uteroplacental Insufficiency (UPI)

Uteroplacental insufficiency occurs when the blood flow, and consequently oxygen supply, from mother to foetus is impaired or inadequate in some way. This is usually the result of an acute or chronic maternal illness (e.g. hypertension, diabetes, pre-eclampsia, kidney disease), although it can arise from chromosomal abnormalities in the foetus. It may also occur in cases of multiple gestation (i.e. twins, triplets or more).

With UPI, steps are taken to correct or treat the underlying cause. Foetal distress may be cause for immediate Caesarean delivery.

Placenta Previa

A placenta that implants and grows near or covering the cervical opening, or os, occurs in up to 20 per cent of pregnancies in the second trimester. This condition, called placenta previa, often resolves itself by moving upward and away from the os about 90 per cent of the time. However, if placenta previa persists late in pregnancy, potentially life-threatening haemorrhage can occur when the cervix starts to efface (thin) if the placenta separates prematurely.

Placenta previa may be total (completely covering the os), partial (partially covering the os) or marginal (on the margin or edge of the os). The condition is diagnosed by ultrasound. Vaginal bleeding is a possible symptom, but some women have no symptoms whatsoever.

If bleeding does occur, bed rest may be prescribed. A blood transfusion may also be necessary. Women who have a complete placenta previa will require a Caesarean delivery. Those with a partial or marginal placenta previa can potentially deliver vaginally, but both the patient and the provider should be prepared for an emergency Caesarean if required.

A low-lying placenta is a one that is near the os, but not close enough to be considered marginal. As with placenta previa, this type of placental implantation has a higher risk of separation during late pregnancy.

Placental Abruption

Vaginal bleeding, abdominal cramp and symptoms of shock (irregular heartbeat, low blood pressure, pale complexion) can signal that the placenta has begun to prematurely separate from the wall of the uterus, a condition called placental abruption (or *abruptio placenta*). Risk factors for placental abruption include maternal high blood pressure, cocaine use or physical trauma to the abdomen.

Abruption may occur anytime after week 20, and if you have had a previous occurrence in an earlier pregnancy, your risk of experiencing it again is increased. Placental abruption may cause major life-threatening haemorrhage, foetal distress or possibly death, and preterm labour. However, a swift diagnosis and initiation of treatment, including blood transfusion, IV fluids and oxygen, can do much to improve outcomes. Immediate delivery, possibly by Caesarean, will be indicated in the majority of cases, but depends on the stability of both mother and foetus and the length of gestation.

Placenta Accreta

Placenta accreta occurs when the placenta implants or attaches to the myometrium, or uterine muscle, instead of the endometrium. Placenta accreta can be further categorized into two subtypes based on the extent of myometrium invasion – placenta increta and placenta percreta.

In pregnancy complicated by placenta accreta, the placenta does not easily separate from the uterine wall during the third stage of delivery, and haemorrhage occurs. A postpartum blood transfusion, arterial embolization or an emergency hysterectomy (surgical removal of the uterus) may be required to stop the bleeding and stabilize the patient. If you are diagnosed with this condition prior to delivery, it's important to discuss the possibility of a hysterectomy. In some clinical situations, a hysterectomy may be unavoidable, but if an option is available, your doctor needs to know of any desire for more children so he can preserve your fertility if at all possible.

Placenta accreta is more likely to occur in women with a history of Caesarean delivery (and climbs with each subsequent Caesarean). In addition, women diagnosed with placenta previa in previous pregnancies have a greatly increased risk of placenta accreta.

tips

If you are considered at risk for the condition, magnetic resonance imaging (MRI) and ultrasound may be used to confirm a diagnosis. A high alpha-foetoprotein (AFP) level may also be a sign of placenta accreta. See Chapter 5 for more details on these diagnostic tests.

Pre-eclampsia/Toxaemia/Eclampsia

Pregnancy-induced hypertension (PIH), or otherwise uncomplicated high blood pressure of pregnancy, mainly occurring after 24 weeks gestation, appears in up to 10 per cent of pregnancies. A condition called pre-eclampsia (or toxaemia) happens in 7 per cent of pregnancies and is characterized by the following symptoms:

- High blood pressure
- Excessive swelling of hands and/or feet
- Sudden weight gain
- Protein in the urine
- Blurred vision
- Abdominal pain
- Headache

Pre-eclampsia may be controlled by bed rest, medication and careful monitoring of the foetus. Hospitalization may be required. If the pregnancy has reached 37 weeks, delivery may be induced or performed via Caesarean to avoid further risk.

When pre-eclampsia does not improve with treatment, or remains undiagnosed, it may develop into eclampsia, a rare but potentially life-threatening condition where convulsions occur.

Premature Labour

Delivery of your baby after week 24 and before week 37 of pregnancy is considered preterm or premature. In cases of very early preterm labour where foetal lung maturity hasn't been established, your doctor will probably try to delay the delivery for as long as possible. Premature babies can suffer from a wide range of physical, neurological and developmental difficulties, so any extra time spent in the womb is beneficial.

Are You At Risk?

A number of environmental and physical factors can increase your chance of preterm delivery. These include, but are not limited to:

· Previous premature labour
· Pregnant with multiples (twins or more)
· Previous uterine surgery
· Hypertension (high blood pressure)
· Cigarette smoking
· Diagnosed incompetent cervix
· Drug or alcohol abuse
· Vaginal or systemic infection
· Exposure to drug diethylstilbestrol (DES)
· Preterm, premature rupture of membranes (PPROM)

Warning Signs

If you experience any of the following warning signs of preterm labour, call your doctor immediately. If you are unable to get in touch with her for any reason, go directly to the nearest hospital emergency department. With prompt action, it may be possible to delay your labour until your unborn child has adequate time to develop.
Symptoms include:

· Painful contractions at regular intervals
· Abdominal cramp
· Lower backache
· Bloody vaginal discharge
· Stomach pain
· Any type of fluid leak from the vagina, large or small

Treatment

Preterm labour may be halted by bed rest, tocolytic medications (drugs that stop contractions) and intravenous hydration. Depending on your medical history and how far along your pregnancy is, you may be hospitalized. Home bed rest may also be prescribed, and you may be required to hook up to a foetal monitor on a regular basis. If preterm labour occurs between 24 and 34 weeks, corticosteroids may be administered to hasten foetal lung surfactant development, as well.

If your cervix dilates to 4 or 5cm (1³/₈–2in), or if your foetus is showing signs of distress, preterm delivery may be unavoidable.

A level-three neonatal intensive care unit (NICU) is the best place for your newborn to receive treatment if he or she is delivered preterm. These units are highly experienced in the care of high-risk newborns and preemies and have state-of-the-art technology and training. Although this is a highly stressful situation, try to remember that everyone is doing their best for your baby. For more information on spending time in the NICU, see Chapter 7.

Preterm Premature Rupture of Membranes (PPROM)

Premature rupture of the amniotic membrane is not necessarily a problem if it occurs late in pregnancy. However, when it happens before week 37 of gestation, certain steps should be taken to ensure that your foetus has enough time for development in the womb.

PPROM may occur in women at risk of preterm labour. Other possible causes of PPROM include cervical incompetence and vaginal infection. If PPROM occurs prior to 37 weeks, bed rest and frequent foetal heart monitoring may be undertaken in an effort to prolong pregnancy until the foetal lungs mature. Antibiotics are administered to ward off infection in both foetus and mother, and steroids may be prescribed to speed lung surfactant production in the foetus.

Bed Rest

If you're experiencing a medical condition that puts you at risk for preterm labour, your doctor may send you to your room for strict bed rest.

Why Bed Rest May Be Necessary

Bed rest takes the forces of gravity off your cervix, gives your circulatory system and blood pressure a break, and has the added benefit of promoting rest and stress reduction.

Amniotic fluid that is greenish or brown in colour may contain meconium, your baby's first bowel movement. The presence of meconium can indicate foetal distress, as the tarry substance may be aspirated (inhaled) in the womb. If you are leaking amniotic fluid and there are signs of meconium, the situation should be evaluated by your doctor immediately.

Staying Sane

At first, that bed may seem like a welcome oasis, particularly if you've been getting little sleep of late. A prescription to snooze! What more could you ask for?

That feeling will probably be short-lived, however. There's only so much you can do horizontally (or even slightly tilted). Yet there are ways to make the time pass a little faster. Some ideas to keep busy beyond the usual TV and hired video fare:

· **Baby shopping by mail or modem**. Get on your laptop or leaf through some of those catalogues you have been inundated with. Shopping has never been so easy on your feet.
· **Get crafty.** Creating something special for baby – embroidered, crocheted or knitted – is a good way to pass the hours. Even if you are a novice, a beginner's kit can get you started. You may not have the time again for years, so go for it.
· **Feed your mind.** Read, read, read. Not just baby books (although feel free to keep this one handy), but classics, new fiction and anything else you can get your hands on.
· **Catch up.** All those pictures you've been meaning to put into photo albums, the scrapbooks that are half finished, letters on your list to

write, and other assorted undertakings are perfect bed-rest projects that have the added bonus of giving a sense of achievement.

· **Be game.** Dust off some of those old board and strategy games you haven't played in years, and recruit your partner or kids to play, too. A rousing game of Risk can be a lot more entertaining than another evening spent channel-hopping.

Miscarriage

Up to 20 per cent of all detected pregnancies miscarry before 20 weeks of gestation. Also referred to as spontaneous abortion or missed abortion, about 50 per cent of miscarriages are thought to be caused by chromosomal abnormalities, or what's known as a blighted ovum – a fertilized egg that implants itself but does not develop into an embryo.

Other factors to be considered in a miscarriage are:
· Hormonal deficiencies
· Abnormalities of the cervix or uterus
· Incompatible blood types or the Rh factor
· Viruses and infections
· Immune disorders

Warning Signs

Some of the warning signs of miscarriage can also happen in perfectly normal and healthy pregnancies. Light blood spotting, for example, is a common occurrence in pregnancy when implantation takes place, and may occur throughout the first trimester.

Better safe than sorry is always the rule in pregnancy, however. Do take any symptoms seriously, and contact your doctor as soon as they occur, but keep in mind that the appearance of blood spots or minor cramp doesn't guarantee miscarriage.

Signs and symptoms of miscarriage may include:
· Bright red vaginal bleeding
· Abdominal cramp

· Low back pain
· High fever
· Extreme nausea and vomiting that's sudden and unusual
· Amniotic fluid leakage
· Severe headache

Some women panic when they experience a sudden improvement in previously troublesome pregnancy symptoms. Remember that this is a common phenomenon toward the end of the first trimester, as hormone levels start to balance out. If you're still concerned, or something just doesn't feel quite right, call your doctor to schedule a quick appointment for a listen to the foetal heartbeat. Most will be happy to comply, if only to ease your mind.

Coping with Loss

It doesn't take long to fall hopelessly in love with your unborn child, to dream about your future together and to start making a special place within your family for him or her. 'Love at first thought' is perhaps the most accurate way to describe how many mums and dads feel about it.

We lost a baby, our first, to miscarriage last year. Is there anything we can do to prevent it this time around?
Many miscarriages occur due to factors completely beyond anyone's control – a defective egg or sperm, implantation outside of the endometrium. Other triggers, such as teratogen exposure, may be avoided with special precautions in pregnancy. Definitely speak to your doctor about your concerns and any special instructions given your medical history (such as activity restrictions).

That is what makes pregnancy loss so difficult at any point in the process. You may hear insensitive comments like, 'Well, at least you were only a few weeks along', that are meant to be sympathetic but only serve to minimize the very real grief you are experiencing. Give yourself adequate time to mourn, and to deal with the feelings of anger, guilt, frustration and depression. Talk to your doctor about a referral to a pregnancy loss support group or a one-to-one counsellor or therapist.

It's extremely important to take care of yourself during this difficult time. If you hadn't yet told anyone about the pregnancy by the time the miscarriage occurred, it may be harder to find enough time to reflect and grieve. Allow yourself to take a few sick or personal days off from work to spend healing time with your partner and family. Don't rush things.

Trying Again

When to try again is a delicate issue. You need to be ready both emotionally and physically. Make sure you have had time to grieve for your loss, and talk to your doctor about the causes behind your first miscarriage. Your doctor might recommend you wait for a while, to allow your body time to recover. If you do want to try again immediately, make sure you express your wishes so you both can prepare properly for the next time.

If you've experienced repeated miscarriages, considered clinically to be three consecutive pregnancy losses before 20 weeks, further investigation will be in order before attempting another pregnancy. The cause can sometimes be determined by a pathological examination of the miscarried foetus or embryo. A meeting with a genetic counsellor and a full pre-conception diagnostic workup to examine your fallopian tubes, uterus and other possible sites of a problem, may also be recommended.

Chapter 14

Month 7

It's the home stretch, the final act, the big countdown – the third trimester. You've made a lot of decisions so far, and there are even more to be made this month. Full speed ahead with labour and delivery preparations this month, as you sign up for childbirth classes and start to assemble a birth plan.

Baby This Month

Weighing in at 1.8kg (4lb) and about 405mm (16in) long, your baby is growing amazingly fast now. Her red, wrinkled skin is losing its fine lanugo covering as more insulating fat accumulates. And her eyelids, closed for so long, can now open and afford her a dim view of the place she will call home for just a few more months.

▲ You and your baby as you start the third trimester.

Dramatic developments in the brain and central nervous system are also occurring, as baby's nerve cells are sheathed with a substance called myelin that speeds nerve impulses. A seven-month-old foetus feels pain, can cry and responds to stimulation from light or sound outside the womb.

Her gymnastics may subside as her space gets smaller, but you're feeling her more intensely now, and her movements may even be visible to both you and your partner. Periodically, tiny elbows and feet will turn your belly into an interactive relief map. Gently pushing back can provide endless entertainment for all three of you. You've heard about it, now play the game at home – it's 'Name That Body Part'.

Even though your foetus is still producing lung surfactant and developing alveoli (air sacs), her lungs still aren't developed enough to breathe in the outside world. If complications required an early delivery now, steroids might be administered intravenously to boost surfactant production. Chemical surfactants can also be used after birth to help with respiratory distress.

Your Body This Month

You're probably feeling perpetually stuffed and slightly out of breath as your uterus relocates all your internal organs. The relief and energy felt in the second trimester may start to fade now. Just remember, you're almost there!

Your Body Changes

The top of the fundus is halfway between your belly button and your breastbone, displacing your stomach, intestines and diaphragm. Your expanding abdomen has formed a shelf, handy for resting your arms on and balancing a cold drink at the cinema. On the downside, you'll be catching a lot of crumbs, and your napkin just doesn't seem to stay on your lap anymore.

Not only are your breasts heavier, but also they are more glandular and getting ready to feed your baby. In this last trimester, your nipples may begin to leak colostrum, which is the yellowish, nutrient-rich fluid that precedes real breast milk. You may find the leaking more apparent when you're sexually aroused. To reduce backaches and breast tenderness, make sure you wear a well-fitting bra (even in bed if it helps). If you are planning on breast-feeding, you may want to consider buying some supportive nursing bras now that can take you through the rest of pregnancy and right into the postpartum period.

If you're buying nursing bras, make sure to test-drive the clasps for easy nursing access. Try to unfasten and slip the nursing flaps down with one hand. This may seem unimportant now, but when you're in the middle of a crowded shopping centre juggling packages and trying to discreetly put baby to breast single-handedly, you'll be thankful you had the foresight.

What You Feel Like

Your body is warming up for labour, and you may start to experience Braxton-Hicks contractions. These painless and irregular contractions feel as if your uterus is making a fist and then gradually relaxing it. If your little one is fairly active, you may think that she is stretching herself sideways at first. A check of your belly may reveal a visible tightening.

Braxton-Hicks contractionscan begin as early as week 20 and continue right up until your due date, although they're more commonly felt in the final month of pregnancy. Some first-time mums-to-be are afraid they won't be able to tell the difference between Braxton-Hicks and actual labour contractions. As any woman who has been through labour will attest, when the real thing comes you'll know it. Rule of thumb: if it hurts, it's labour.

Starting at week 20, the uterus has a basic rhythm. The smooth muscle of the uterus is similar to your intestinal tract, in that both involuntarily contract in a wavelike pattern designed to facilitate movement of what's inside (be it breakfast or your baby). These early rhythmic and generally painless contractions are called Braxton-Hicks when they do not cause any changes to the cervix and occur at irregular intervals. They may even be uncomfortable at times, but will usually subside if you change positions, another way to distinguish Braxton-Hicks from the real thing. The actual definition of labour, even when it is premature, is the onset of regular, painful, uterine contractions that lead to a change in the cervix.

If your contractions suddenly seem to be coming at regular intervals and start to cause you pain or discomfort, they may be the real thing. Lie down on your left side for about a half-hour with a clock or watch on hand, and time the contractions from the beginning of one to the beginning of the next. If the interludes are more or less regular, call your doctor. And if contractions of any type are accompanied by blood or amniotic fluid leakage, contact your doctor immediately.

The list is growing – other symptoms that may continue this month include:

- Fatigue
- Frequent urination
- Tender and/or swollen breasts
- Bleeding gums
- Excess mucus and saliva
- Increase in normal vaginal discharge
- Mild shortness of breath
- Lightheadedness or dizziness
- Headaches
- Forgetfulness
- Wind, heartburn and/or constipation
- Skin and hair changes
- Round ligament pain or soreness
- Lower back aches
- Mild swelling of legs, feet and hands
- Leg cramp

At the Doctor

Your doctor will probably want to know if you've been experiencing any Braxton-Hicks contractions, and he will cover the warning signs of preterm labour and what you should do if you experience them (see Chapter 13). If you're unsure about what type of childbirth class is available, you might want to ask your doctor for her opinion. Just remember, the decision is ultimately up to you and your partner.

Women who are Rh negative will need treatment with Rh immune globulin (RhoGAM) this month. An injection is typically given at about 28 weeks to protect the foetus from developing haemolytic disease – a condition where the mother's antibodies attack the foetal red blood cells.

Why is everyone always touching me, and how can I get them to stop?

People are fascinated with the life force of pregnancy, and you're radiating it big-time. While your family is granted fairly open access to your belly, colleagues and acquaintances are another story. To fend off the feelers who ask permission first, simply tell them you're sensitive about your stomach right now. You may have a tougher time stopping those swoopers who strike without warning, but if you can anticipate their moves you might be able to block with a step back or a turn away. Hopefully, they'll get the hint.

On Your Mind

This month will bring new questions and uncertainties as you ponder your ideal birth experience. Are you looking forward to a completely chemical-free birth, or are you already exploring your pain-killing options? Is your doctor open to your needs and willing to make reasonable accommodation to meet them? Do you want only your partner in attendance, or would you like additional support? Whatever your perfect labour and delivery may be, make sure the direction of your birth plan is driven by the needs of yourself and your partner, and not by the expectations of others.

Keep in mind that you don't want to create such incredibly high expectations of yourself and of the experience that you're bound to be let down. Try to build in room for flexibility in your conception of the ultimate birth. Your little one may not be following the same game plan as you, and last-minute strategy changes are often required. Luckily, if you work on your birth plan now, you will be able to make allowances for complications within it and save yourself unnecessary angst later.

Childbirth Classes

Most childbirth seminars available through hospitals and birth centres use lectures, audiovisuals and floor exercises to get you ready for labour and delivery. They may vary in length from several months of Saturdays to a one-day seminar. While hospital policy will dictate a lot of what's covered, here's a general idea of what you will experience:

- **Commiseration.** You'll interact with other pregnant couples and demonstrate that misery (and joy) truly does love company.
- **Reality.** Through lecture and (in many cases) actual video footage, you'll get the full view on what really goes on in labour and delivery.
- **Guided tour.** If your class is at the birth centre or hospital, you will probably get a tour of the facilities and some basic instructions on when and where to show up when labour hits. The best part? The nursery window stop, of course.
- **Teamwork.** Your husband, partner or birth companion will learn more about his or her role in this process, and you may even be given homework to try out techniques at home.
- **After-birth instruction.** Many classes offer valuable information on breast-feeding basics and baby care. Don't be surprised if the instructor brings in a bag full of baby dolls for practice.
- **Seasoned support.** Most prepared childbirth classes will be conducted by a trained childbirth educator.
- **Paperwork.** More literature, brochures, pamphlets, handouts, forms, photocopies and leaflets will come your way. Bring a bag.

Perhaps the most important facet of childbirth class, and certainly the one that most first-time mums pay the closest attention to, is the information it provides on managing labour and delivery discomforts. In addition to an overview of anesthesia and pain medication options, childbirth educators may draw on one or more childbirth philosophies to teach coping methods. Some of the most popular and widely taught techniques are outlined below.

Lamaze Method

Lamaze, or psychoprophylaxis, is probably the most well-known childbirth method in use in the United States today. Named after Dr Fernand Lamaze, classes are taught by certified Lamaze instructors and attended by more than 2,000,000 parents-to-be annually.

If you've never been in a Lamaze class, you probably equate the name with heavy, hyperventilated breathing. True Lamaze classes, however, are much more than panting practice. While rhythmic breathing exercises are stressed for each stage of labour in Lamaze, helpful labouring and birth positions, relaxation techniques and pain management are also covered. In addition to massage, water therapy and hot and cold compresses, you're taught how to focus on a picture or object to diminish your discomfort.

Lamaze is founded on the principle that instinct and what Lamaze International calls 'inner wisdom' guide women through the birth process. Lamaze also stresses the empowerment of the mother-to-be and her right to the birth experience and environment she wants.

Bradley Method

Denver obstetrician Robert Bradley, the author of *Husband-Coached Childbirth,* developed this popular approach to labour and delivery. As you may have guessed, he was a big advocate of fathers helping their partners through the birth process, and in fact many consider his work instrumental in opening up the labour room door to dads.

Bradley classes teach couples how to relax and breathe deeply, but the emphasis is on doing what comes naturally – father as coach, proper nutrition during pregnancy and, most importantly, knowing all the options beforehand. They also emphasize the *natural* in natural childbirth, suggesting that pain medication be used as a last resort, rather than a front-line tool.

Hypnobirthing and Dr Grantly Dick-Read

Doctor and natural childbirth pioneer Grantly Dick-Read, who wrote the classic *Childbirth Without Fear,* is the inspiration behind hypnobirthing education. Dick-Read believed that a woman's labour pains were magnified by her fears and anxieties. Hypnobirthing, based on Dick-Read's teachings, emphasizes slow abdominal breathing and other relaxation techniques that teach you how to focus on the feelings and signals your body sends during labour.

LeBoyer Method

Dr Frederick LeBoyer, author of *Birth Without Violence*, developed this method of childbirth that attempts to soften the trauma of the transition from the warm, dark womb to the big bright world. It advocates dim lights in the delivery room, a warm bath for the new baby, calm voices and soothing room temperatures.

If your last pregnancy ended in a Caesarean section and you're going to try to deliver vaginally this time around, inquire about a VBAC, or vaginal birth after caesarean, class. VBAC courses provide couples with information on the benefits, risks and statistics surrounding vaginal births following a Caesarean. They are usually recommended as a supplement to, and not a replacement for, a prepared childbirth class.

The Right Teacher and the Right Class

Completely confused now? Don't know your Bradley from your LeBoyer? A good first step is to call your hospital or birth centre and ask for printed schedules and descriptions of coming classes – many of your questions will probably be answered there. Once you get a basic feel for what is offered, you can call with follow-up questions about instructor credentials and training, methods taught, class size, curriculum and costs. You might also ask if there are couples who have taken the course that you can contact as references.

If you find that the classes offered at your local hospital just aren't what you're looking for, you may opt for private classes. Ask your caregiver for advice, or contact the Natural Childbirth Trust at www.nct-online.org.

Touring the Hospital/Birth Centre

Even if you don't choose a childbirth class sponsored by the facility at which you'll be giving birth, you should try to arrange a tour. Getting your bearings ahead of time will save you valuable time and frustration when the big day arrives. If you're in the middle of the mother of -all contractions, the last thing you want to do is try to figure out where visitor parking is. You'll also have less anxiety and disappointment if you know what to expect of the labour and birth rooms. What you imagine (a flower-filled, sunny room filled with soft music and framed watercolours) may be a far cry from reality.

Just for Dads

Depending on today's viewpoint, the light, or the fire, at the end of the tunnel is becoming brighter. In three months you will be witnessing your child's first breath in this world. Although your partner will be doing the really hard work, you'll need to start studying your role in this final drama as (A) a shoulder to lean on; (B) a forgiving target to vent at; and (C) head cheerleader.

About Childbirth Classes

If you are the type that thrives on clear instructions and routine, you may find the idea of childbirth class a port in the pregnancy storm. 'Hooray!' you think, 'At last someone is going to tell me what to do.' Well, not quite. Yes, you will be taught techniques you can use to help your partner through labour and delivery, and you'll learn in graphic detail just how that baby is going to get from point A to point B. But you aren't getting any step-by-step instructions or checklists that are money-back guaranteed to get you from the first contraction to 'It's a boy/girl!' Labour and delivery is not a maths problem or a computer program. Your best preparation is to be ready for the unexpected.

fact

Second, third or fourth time around? There are benefits in taking a childbirth class for even the most experienced parents. First of all, most instructors stay updated on the latest developments in obstetrical medicine, so if there's something new under the sun in labour and delivery, the class is the place to learn about it. And from an altruistic viewpoint, other first-time parents will jump at the chance to hear about birth from seasoned pros. If scheduling is an issue, many facilities offer less time-intensive 'brush-up' courses for veterans of the pregnancy wars.

Don't think of the class as... well, class, either. It is an educational experience, but you aren't being graded on your performance. In other words, if academia is not your strong point, you don't need to be in a panic. The only background you need to succeed in childbirth class is a willingness to learn and listen, and a pregnant partner. There will be no sudden quizzes here.

Putting on the Birth Partner's Hat

Lesson number one: being a birth partner is being supportive, helping your partner learn about birth as she progresses through labour, giving her the tools she needs to get her through the rough spots and, above all, providing positive reinforcement and encouragement.

You likely don't need to be told this, but barking orders at your partner (assuming you would have the seriously misguided courage to do so) will get you nowhere but kicked out of the room. You'll learn much more about your role as birth partner in prepared childbirth class, but you may want to turn ahead to Chapter 18 for a preview now.

Chapter 15

Blueprint for Birth: Writing Your Birth Plan

A birth plan is a road map for your entire childbirth experience, beginning to end. It's your chance to let everyone involved (doctors, nurses, partners) know what you want the experience to be. Use it to chart the course of labour and delivery, but remember you may have to take alternate routes occasionally, depending on conditions.

Why Have a Birth Plan?

The process of talking through and creating a birth plan helps you and your partner establish what you want out of childbirth (apart from the child, of course). Having it down as written words can ease your anxieties about labour and delivery. And when things go crazy as the big day arrives, a birth plan can be your calm in the storm, something solid to grasp when you suddenly seem to have forgotten just about everything you've learned.

A birth plan also serves the very important purpose of letting your doctor know just what kind of experience and level of intervention you're looking for. Because it can tread on some sensitive and controversial medical territory, it's important that you include your doctor or midwife in the process.

Preparing Your Provider

Once you and your partner have put your birth plan together, you should present it to your doctor for his comments and questions. Communicating your wishes and being receptive to feedback can make the difference between a birth plan that works and one that doesn't.

Many doctors and midwives will set up a separate visit dedicated to discussing the birth plan you've come up with. Consider the plan you take to him or her initially a first draft. You can then incorporate your doctor's input into your final plan.

Once you have reviewed your birth plan with your doctor, ask her to place a copy in your chart and hospital record. Make sure everyone else who will be present at the birth has one as well, so everyone is working to the same game plan.

Unfortunately, not all doctors are thrilled about the prospect of a birth plan. They can be a difficult issue for some doctors, who don't like to feel that their patients don't trust them; or don't want to have a disappointed patient if the actual birth strays from the plan. For these reasons, birth plans have the potential to set up an adversarial feeling in some doctor-patient relationships.

How can you prevent your birth plan from becoming a bone of contention? First, be willing to really listen to any suggestions or issues your doctor has, and make an effort to work toward a resolution together. Also, try to keep your expectations grounded in reality and not over restrictive. Wanting your three-year-old to be nearby so she can meet her sibling shortly after birth is great, but insisting she be on the spot the moment the baby's head emerges is unrealistic.

Make It User-Friendly

If you hand your midwife a birth plan the size of *War and Peace*, she might start to wonder what she's got herself into. While covering all your options is important, you simply can't control every possible aspect of what may or may not occur during labour and delivery. Medical emergencies do happen, which is why you have a doctor or midwife to begin with. You need to trust your doctor to follow the *spirit* of your birth plan, while making adjustments for the health of you and your baby. Establishing a good, communicative relationship is the best way to ensure this.

Conciseness is better from a logistical viewpoint, too. The medical staff attending your birth and aftercare should be able to easily access and reference the information. Think brevity and bullet points, and keep it under five pages, if possible; fewer than that is even better.

Try to use language that is co-operative and communicative. Your birth plan should not read like a ransom note. Filling it with demands and absolutes leaves your doctor very little room to make appropriate medical suggestions should the birth go off-course.

The bottom line is that labour is very unpredictable, and rarely do birth plans get followed to the letter. Outlining your wishes in terms of preferences, and giving your doctor or midwife alternatives in case complications arise, will make your birth plan more useful to everyone involved, especially you and baby.

Atmosphere

Comfortable surroundings will help both your mind and body relax during labour. Whether you're giving birth in a hospital, at home or somewhere in between, outlining your preference for what you'll be seeing and hearing around you is an important component of the birth plan.

The Perfect Place

First, know what you have to work with. Hospital birth facilities are starting to recognize the value of a pleasant, warm atmosphere. You may find yours is already set up to suit your needs well.

However, if things look a little sterile and spartan, there are ways to make it more welcoming. Easy and acceptable additions include a cozy blanket and pillow from home, a picture or two (which may serve double duty as focal points during contractions) and fresh flowers. You may also be able to adjust the lights and sounds to make things more relaxing.

Home birth may also be an option if you feel strongly about giving birth in familiar surroundings and among family. However, home birth doesn't mean you should opt out of a health-care professional's help; in fact, it's even more important, since you won't have access to the medical monitoring and diagnostic equipment that a hospital offers. In many uncomplicated pregnancies, a home birth can be a completely safe and emotionally rewarding choice; however, women who may experience high-risk deliveries for any reason need to seriously contemplate the benefits and safety of a hospital birth.

An in-between alternative for some women might be a birth centre, which is equipped to handle some medical problems that may occur yet can offer less conventional labour and delivery methods, such as a water birth.

Music and Lighting

Music is one of the easiest ways to change the mood. Just bring a portable stereo and a few diverse musical selections in case you need a change of pace, and you're all set. Classical music may help to soothe and centre you, and something fast and furious can get the adrenaline going for the hard work. Just be conscious of the fact that other mums are likely to be in labour nearby, and your baby is not wearing earplugs. Keep the volume down, or use headphones if you don't mind yet another line connecting you to something.

As far as lighting goes, you may not have a lot of choices beyond off/on if you're giving birth in a hospital setting. Even if you can dim the lights, you want your doctor or midwife to be able to see what she's doing. But requesting that the curtains are drawn and the lights turned down during early and active labour is not unreasonable.

Photo Finish

Chances are you will want pictures, and lots of them. Your birth plan can outline your audiovisual expectations (video of the delivery, pictures of a Caesarean in the operating room, live Web cast of baby's first breath). It also serves as a good checklist for you and your partner when packing for the hospital.

If you want to capture your little star's debut on video, it's best to check with your doctor to make sure there's no policy against an amateur videographer being underfoot. Even if there is, in some cases you may be able to work out a compromise, such as setting up the camera in advance on a stationary tripod.

Family, Friends and Support

So who will be at the big event? This is perhaps one of the most crucial parts of a birth plan, to prepare for adequate support during this very difficult job that lies ahead. Is this a personal experience for just you and your partner, or do you want additional family, friends or other support there? It's even harder for first-time mums, who may have misconceptions about exactly what will happen and who will be there when they hit the maternity ward.

Many women think that their doctor, midwife or, at least, a dedicated staff nurse, will be available to assist them with the entire labour and birth. In most places, that simply isn't true for a variety of reasons. Shift changes, the number of patients in labour and other factors may have you and your partner spending a lot of time alone. Having a birth companion on your labour team is a great way to ensure continuity of care.

Why enlist a companion if a dad is present? Many companions will provide early labour support at home, a benefit that most doctor's can't match. It's also reassuring to many dads to know that they have a back-up, and aren't forced to remember everything they learned in their six-week childbirth class during this time. If you are being cared for by a domino system, you will have a familiar midwife with you throughout the birth

If you will have people waiting at the hospital who won't be participating in your birth but who you would like to introduce to the baby as soon as possible, indicate this in the birth plan. And don't forget about a minder for young children, who need supervision and support.

Getting Ready

You have the people and the place set. Now for some decisions that will affect your comfort and mobility during labour.

Food and Drink

Some hospitals and providers put a strict ban on eating during labour for several reasons. First, if things don't go as planned and you end up having a general anesthetic for a Caesarean, having food in your stomach puts you at risk for aspiration (inhaling vomit). Second, your stomach and gastrointestinal tract will have to digest that food, when clearly there is more important action happening right next door.

That said, labour lasts a very long time for many women, who may need some sustenance. Simple, liquid-based carbohydrates such as a glass of juice, ice lolly or juice bar, broth, or tea or lemonade with honey are easily digested and may give you a boost. Outline what you'd like to have access to so you can discuss it with your doctor. If your doctor or hospital believes a light snack of food and drink is an absolute no-no in labour, intravenous lines will probably be used to take care of any risk of dehydration. However, a dry mouth is annoying and uncomfortable, so see if you can at least get ice cubes to suck on, and bring your lip balm.

Monitors and Mobility

Being tethered to a bed can make handling contractions and labour difficult. Yet checking the foetal heart rate and your contractions is important to ensure baby isn't encountering any stress. To give yourself room to move through the contractions while ensuring your little one's safety, ask for intermittent monitoring. Unless you require internal monitoring, which is sometimes the case in higher-risk pregnancies, having the freedom to move at least part of the time shouldn't be an issue. Newer wireless foetal monitors may let you cut the cord altogether.

▲ A foetal monitor can assess your baby's heart rate and check for signs of foetal distress.

Pain Relief

One of the biggest decisions of childbirth is whether you will want, or need, pharmaceutical pain relief. Chapter 18 has a full assessment of your labour and delivery pain relief options. Your doctor or midwife and anesthesiologist can also shed more light on the use of painkillers .

Going Natural

If you intend to go completely drug-free, this section of your birth plan may be a bit more detailed. You'll want to outline the access you'd like to other, drug-free pain relief strategies. Things like hydrotherapy (shower or whirlpool), massage and birth balls or a TENS machine may be on your list. Requesting to go natural doesn't close the door on changing your mind. If you're a first-time mum, you can't predict whether pain medication will be necessary.

A birth ball is a large, inflatable heavy-gauge rubber ball that you can sit on, drape yourself over or do just about anything else with that feels comfortable during a contraction. The balls are available in different sizes, and some even come in oblong or ridged versions if you're concerned about tipping over. When used in the sitting position, the natural give of the ball may encourage perineal relaxation.

Timing of Pain Relief

Some doctors and midwives may have policies about how late, or how early, in labour they will permit an epidural. Whether their policy is grounded in research, experience or preference will probably make the difference in whether they are willing to be flexible on this point. If you have strong feelings about when you want access to an epidural or other pain relief option, outline your wishes in your birth plan.

When to Change Course: Interventions

Your doctor will warn you up front that unforeseen circumstances may mean a deviation from your birth plan. Sometimes women feel as if they have failed if things do not go precisely according to their concept of the ideal birth – which is certainly not the case. The best way to avoid disappointment is to build alternative scenarios into your birth plan regarding interventions that might be required. For example, if you really don't want an episiotomy, you should indicate that in your birth plan, and suggest perineal massage with vitamin E oil or another lubricant, warm compresses or another acceptable alternative. But be prepared to work with your doctor during labour if your alternative plan just doesn't do the trick. And don't be too prescriptive – when you start instructing your physician in the type of sutures to use, you're forgetting that he's there because of his medical expertise, not in spite of it.

Some possible interventions that may come up in labour and delivery include:

- Induction
- Forceps use
- Vacuum extraction
- Episiotomy
- Artificial membrane rupture
- Labour augmentation (via the drug oxytocin, or Pitocin)

Other Considerations

The choices continue after labour and delivery, and include decisions not just about your care, but also about the care of your new son or daughter.

I'm having a Caesarean. Why bother with a birth plan?
As you can see, a birth plan encompasses much more than baby's passage from point A to point B. Even with a Caesarean birth, there are many choices along the way. For example, will dad be in the delivery room? Does he want to cut the cord? Can video be taken? Will you get to spend time with your baby right after the procedure? Because things can be a little more rigid rule-wise in the environment of an operating room, these are important issues to clear with your doctor ahead of time. A birth plan will help you do just that.

Cutting the Cord

You or your partner may be given the option to cut the baby's umbilical cord if you want to. Keep in mind that if your baby needs immediate medical attention at birth, it's possible the cord will be cut swiftly by the attending doctor or midwife instead.

The issue of when exactly to cut the cord may require some negotiations if you have strong feelings about delaying it. If your provider disagrees and believes a swift snip is in order, find out the reasons and research behind his opinion so you can explore the issue further and come to a meeting of the minds, if possible. For more on cutting the umbilical cord, see Chapter 18.

First Contact

Every woman wants her first encounter with her baby to be just perfect. After all, you've had a nine-month build-up to this moment, so wanting to stage and execute it seamlessly is natural.

If you're giving birth in a hospital, find out if there are strict procedures that must be followed with the baby's care immediately following the birth. Will you be able to nuzzle with her for as long as you'd like, or will she be whisked away for cleaning and the rest after a quick hello? Will your other children be able to meet her immediately, or will they have to wait until visiting hours? Contact the hospital before you create this part of your plan so you aren't in for an immediate letdown if your wishes for the first meeting are against hospital policy. If you find the policies are just too restrictive, you still have time to explore other options for where you deliver.

Creative thinking may be required to make some rules and regulations acceptable to you. If you can only hold your baby for a few minutes before she goes for her after-birth tune-up, perhaps your partner can assist with those duties and use this special time to bond with baby.

I don't want my baby getting a bottle or dummy in the hospital. Is it bad form to be so petty in the birth plan?
Not at all. It's actually helpful information to include. While your nurse will probably ask you about your feeding preferences, having it in the chart makes it easier for all involved. If you're planning on breast-feeding and want to ensure that your baby and you establish both a good technique and milk flow in those early days, it's a good idea.

Postpartum Planning

Adding a postpartum section to your birth plan can be tremendous help in getting organized after you and your baby are back at home. Will you have live-in help for a few days or weeks? Are you and your partner both taking time off? Will baby have a whirlwind schedule of introductions to friends and family, or just a few exclusive engagements?

Outline your maternity leave timetable, if you know what it is, and tentative plans for after it's over. Include baby's two-week doctor's visit, so you won't forget to schedule it when he arrives.

Even though your doctor won't need to put his stamp of approval on this portion of your plans, it's a good idea to run them by him. He can give you feedback on whether you'll be physically capable of doing what you've set out to do, to ensure that you have a sufficient recovery period.

Appendix A in the back of this book includes a checklist you can use for guidance in creating your birth plan.

Chapter 16

Month 8

You are a pregnancy pro now, deftly handling all the aches and pains that come with the territory. Even if you've sailed through pregnancy feeling just fine, you've learned to adjust to the fashion hardships, the lifestyle changes and the logistical challenges that your baby and belly have brought to the forefront. It's not much longer now.

Baby This Month

Gradually shifting to the same position in which 95 per cent of all babies are born, your foetus starts to move into a head-down pose, known as the vertex position. The small but stubborn percentage that don't assume the vertex position are considered breech. Feel a lot of kicking on your pelvic floor? It may be a clue that baby is still standing, or sitting, tall. She may also be lounging in the transverse position, or sideways in the womb.

▲ You and your baby in month 8 of gestation.

Your little girl or boy is now up to 460mm (18in) long and as heavy as a 2.2kg (5lb) bag of flour. The rest of her body is finally catching up to the size of her head. Although it may feel as if she's constantly up and about, she's actually sleeping for 90–95 per cent of the day, a figure that will drop only slightly when she is born.

If your child were to be born today, she'd have an excellent chance of surviving and eventually thriving outside the womb. However, she'd still officially be considered preterm or premature, just as any birth before 37 weeks of gestation.

Your Body This Month

Can you still remember your pre-pregnancy body? The little things – like being able to zip up your coat, wear your rings and sit on the floor without requiring adult assistance to stand again – may be a distant memory. You will not be pregnant forever, of course, although it may sometimes feel like it.

If you've been dribbling urine just about every time you sneeze, you're probably experiencing stress incontinence. But if you have a steady leak that seems to be unrelated to bodily stress, it may be amniotic fluid. Amniotic fluid is clear to straw-coloured and has a faintly sweet smell. Less commonly, it may be tinged green or brown. If you think you're leaking amniotic fluid, no matter how small the amount, contact your doctor. If your membranes have ruptured, you risk infection if you don't deliver soon.

Your Body Changes

Weight gain should start to slow down this month. If it doesn't, however, don't cut your calorie intake to try and stop it. You need the extra energy for both of you.

As baby settles firmly on your bladder, toilet breaks step up once again. You may even experience some stress incontinence, which is minor dribbling or leakage of urine when you sneeze, cough, laugh or make other sudden movements. This will clear up postpartum. In the meantime, keep doing your pelvic floor exercises (see Chapter 8), don't hold it in, and wear a pantyliner.

What You Feel Like

Your Weeble-like physique has you off-balance and generally clumsy. Be careful – you wobble and you *can* fall down. And, of course, those (say it together, everyone) pregnancy hormones have loosened up your joints and relaxed your muscles to make you a bit of a butterfingers.

Now is not the ideal time to be fitted for new contact lenses or glasses. Pregnancy-related fluid retention can actually change the shape of your eyes and trigger minor vision changes. Also at work is oestrogen, which causes your eyes to be drier than normal and may make contact lenses uncomfortable now. Unless you want to invest in new eyewear yet again postpartum, you may want to hold fire for now.

It's easier and easier to get winded as your little one pushes up into your diaphragm. Take it slow, breathe deeply and practise good posture. To ease breathing while you sleep, pile on a few extra pillows or use a foam bed wedge to elevate your head.

Other symptoms that may continue this month include:

·   Fatigue
·   Frequent urination
·   Tender and/or swollen breasts
·   Colostrum discharge from nipples
·   Bleeding gums
·   Excess mucus and saliva
·   Increase in normal vaginal discharge
·   Mild shortness of breath
·   Lightheadedness or dizziness
·   Headaches
·   Forgetfulness
·   Wind, heartburn and/or constipation
·   Skin and hair changes
·   Round ligament pain or soreness
·   Lower back aches

- Mild swelling of legs, feet and hands
- Leg cramp
- Painless, irregular contractions (Braxton-Hicks)

If you experience blurred vision or visual disturbances (e.g. spots) and you have high blood pressure or diabetes, let your doctor know immediately. This could be a sign of poor control in both cases, which is dangerous to both you and your child.

At the Doctor

Your provider will check the position of your baby to determine if he has turned head down in preparation for birth.

If your practitioner brings up the possibility of a breech (bottom or foot-first) birth, it's because she or he has felt the head of your unborn baby up near your ribs, or an ultrasound has confirmed that your child is in the breech position. Don't panic. Your fickle foetus is likely to change position again in the next few weeks. If she doesn't, your practitioner may try to turn the baby closer to term, using a technique known as external cephalic version, or manually attempting to turn the foetus in the uterus.

Babies can be delivered vaginally in breech position in some instances, but the procedure is more difficult and carries a higher risk for the infant. It is also not advised for first pregnancies. Caesarean is the method of choice for safe breech delivery. If you really want a vaginal birth and a cephalic version is unsuccessful in turning your breech, some doctors may agree to a trial of labour to see if your contracting uterus helps to turn the child.

External cephalic version (or simply 'version') is successful in turning a breech baby in about half of all instances where it is attempted. However, if it is done too far before the estimated delivery date, there is a possibility that the foetus may flip back to the breech position.

There are three classifications of breech: frank, complete and incomplete. In frank breech, your baby uses your pelvic bone as a seat, and stretches his legs up close to his chest. With incomplete breech, one or both legs will drop down during delivery and will arrive before the rest of the body. This is also called a single- or double-footling breech birth. In a complete breech, your baby has his bottom on your pelvis again, but legs and arms are crossed in front of his little body.

Frank

◀ There are three classifications of breech: frank, complete and incomplete.

Complete (left)
and Incomplete
(right)

On Your Mind

As labour looms closer, your thoughts turn to the task at hand. Going
into labour and delivery with as much knowledge of the process as
possible can make the difference between a positive childbirth experience
and a long and arduous one.

Am I Up to the Task of Labour?

Women have been doing this since the beginning of time, and under
much more difficult circumstances. Yes, in most cases labour will be hard
work, but if you prepare yourself by learning what to expect, you will be
ready to face whatever comes your way. You'll also find that your partner
or labour partner will be a huge asset in helping you through childbirth.

Am I Up to the Task of Motherhood?

In a word – yes. Great mummies are made, not born. While some parts of mothering will seem to come to you instinctively, practice and trial and error will make up the better part of your parenting education. Use the tools around you – your paediatrician, other mothers and research and reading – to build and sharpen your skills, but listen to your inner voice in the final analysis and application of what you learn.

Things That Make You Go Grrrrr

As pregnancy winds down, your patience goes with it. The belly touchers, advice givers, urban-legend spreaders and comedians seem to be everywhere and completely unaware of the dangerously thin ice they are treading on. Rather than biting heads off, take a deep, deep breath and remind yourself that though insensitive, most are well meaning. In the meantime, photocopy the list of no-no's below for your colleagues and hang it in the staff room – maybe it will sink in.

What if I don't get to the hospital in time?
Every woman has heard stories of impatient babies being born in taxis, but these are the exception rather than the rule. Most women have plenty of time to make it to the hospital safe and sound; the average labour period is 12–14 hours. But if you're concerned, you can take some basic precautions. Work out a route in advance, keep your fuel tank full, and have cash on hand for a cab, just in case your car decides to conk out with the first contraction.

Top ten things not to say to a pregnant woman:

1. Haven't you had that baby yet?
2. Are you still here?
3. Wow, you're HUGE!
4. You really should avoid pain medication when you go into labour – it

will hurt the baby.

5. Labour is hell! Take all the drugs you can get!
6. So how much weight have you gained?
7. You don't mind if we call you at home while you're on maternity leave, do you?
8. Are you having twins?
9. You look terrible – why don't you take a nap?
10. This is your captain speaking. Looks like our take-off has been set back another hour. Please be aware that while we are taxiing, leaving your seat to visit the lavatory is not permitted.

Nesting

Ahhh, nesting – that overwhelming urge to turn everything in your house upside down and rearrange it. Your mad dash to finish the nursery and squirrel away a year's supply of baby wipes is an instinctive reaction to baby's upcoming arrival. You're preparing a safe haven for your little one and assuring yourself that all his needs and wants will be adequately met.

A Space for Baby the First Few Weeks

Keeping baby within arm's length during her first few weeks home will improve your rest and peace of mind. A Moses basket, which is about the size and depth of a baby carriage or pram, may make her feel safer and more secure than the openness of a crib. You can roll it right next to your bed and give those 4 AM feedings with ease. It's also an inexpensive way to bed her down if you're still saving your pennies for the perfect crib.

Your rest will continue to be a priority once baby arrives. If you find that having him next to your bed has you sleeping fitfully and waking up at the slightest sigh or kick, consider changing your sleeping arrangements. Have a baby monitor as back-up (you'll need one anyway) in case you find you need to keep him in his own room so both of you can get adequate sleep.

Stocking Up on Essentials

Don't go crazy buying super-sized cases of baby supplies. You may not like the brand or type you purchase, which leaves you with a lot of unwanted merchandise on your hands. Instead, buy small so you can sample. Once you've decided what works best for you and baby, you can stock up at the warehouse outlet.

Some baby essentials you should have on the shelves prior to her arrival: nappies, wipes, surgical spirit swabs (for her umbilical cord), baby shampoo and soap, nappy rash ointment, waterproof pads (a huge plus for cutting down on laundry), bottles (even if you're breast-feeding, you may pump milk occasionally), a thermometer and infant paracetamol or another fever-reducing product recommended by your paediatrician.

What are the pros and cons of using cloth nappies?
If you're thinking green, cloth nappies have the advantage of not ending up in a landfill site, although they do require additional fossil fuels and water resources to wash. Cost can be an advantage, but it's probably a slight one. When washing them, be sure you have the time and the strength to be doing the laundry daily. If your baby has sensitive skin, you might find cloth less irritating. Like most things in parenting, it's trial and error – have a supply of both types, and see how they work for you.

Just for Dads

Indecision and insecurities may plague you this month as the birth draws nearer, made all the more disturbing by your unfamiliarity with these feelings. Try to conquer your anxieties by accepting your weaknesses and valuing your strengths. And recognize the fact that learning is all part of the experience.

Measuring Up

Whether you aspire to be just like your father, or have sworn to be nothing like him at all, you've got some preconceived notion of just what makes the world's best dad. Beyond your own childhood, your idea of fatherhood has been shaped by many different influences, not the least of which are the impossibly patient patriarchs dramatized on the small screen. But while they're nice to visit, you wouldn't want to live with them. Don't try to measure up to a fantasy figure.

Start with the basics. Promise yourself you'll listen to your child, be there for him and instill a sense of values and moral compass through your actions and your words. Love him. That's what a father does best.

Trying to break the baby name stalemate? If you are set on one name and she on another, consider combinations of the two, or variations with first and middle. Still not agreeing? If you don't want resentments on either side, start from scratch and come up with something new that you both like. Draw on your family tree, ethnic heritage, religious beliefs, heroes and heroines, passions and hobbies and anything else important in your life. Just make sure you consider all possible nicknames, initials and obvious rhyming combinations to spare your child grief later.

Nappy Duty and Other Special Skills

If you're a complete novice at infant care, the best way to pick up knowledge is to go to antenatal or parenting classes. You may feel silly playing with dolls at first, but when you do it in a room full of other grown men following suit, it's easier to take. However, if a class isn't an option for you, and you don't have any babies of family or friends that you can take for a test-drive, it won't take you long to learn once your baby arrives.

You'll have the opportunity to change your newborn during her stay in the hospital, under the watchful eye of a nurse if you so desire. This is a safe environment in which to learn if you're a little wary of your abilities.

Always have a clean nappy ready and to hand before removing the soiled one. This is especially important if you have a boy. The phrase that pays: cover that guy, or get a squirt in the eye. If that doesn't help you remember, the first direct hit will. If you're changing a girl, slide the clean nappy under her as soon as possible after the dirty one is removed (unlike a boy, you probably won't notice the puddle until it's too late). If you have a busybody that likes to get his hands into everything (including his nappy), try giving him a small toy to play with while you do your stuff.

The first bath is always cause for some jitters, but your newborn won't be having anything beyond a sponging off until she's back at home and her cord has fallen off (yes, it's supposed to do that). Tag-teaming with your partner on the baby bathing is a great approach to take until you've built up your confidence level.

Chapter 17

Month 9

The grand finale is approaching. You may feel like you've been waiting forever. But even if you had the time of conception pin-pointed, your baby may decide he needs a little more, or a little less, time to get prepared. Never fear – he or she will arrive sooner or later.

Baby This Month

Your child is putting on about 225g (8oz) per week as he prepares to make his big exit. At delivery, the average British birth weight is 3,000–3,499g (6lb 10oz–7lb 11oz).

▲ A final look at you and your foetus before the big day.

He's fully formed and just waiting for the right time now. If you're having a boy, his testicles have descended and may be visible in any nine-month ultrasound images. His lungs, the last organ system to fully mature, now have an adequate level of surfactant in them to allow breathing outside the womb.

A dark, tarry amalgam of amniotic fluid, skin cells and other foetal waste, is gathering in your baby's intestines. This substance, called meconium, will become the contents of his bowel movements during the first few days of life.

Foetal movement will naturally become less vigorous as you get closer to your due date and the baby is pressed for space, but a healthy baby should still be making his presence known. Your doctor may ask you to count foetal kicks. Pick a typically active time of day for your little one, and start counting his moves. Your doctor will let you know how many movements you should feel in what period of time (usually around 8–10 in a space of two hours). If she seems slow, she may be sleeping. Try drinking a glass of juice to get her going. Call your doctor immediately if baby's movements are notably decreased or absent.

Your Body This Month

While baby is still growing, your weight gain tapers off and you may even lose 454g (1lb) or so due to a drop in amniotic fluid production. Groin soreness and backaches are more persistent as the musculoskeletal system strains to support your abdomen. The good news – you can't get any bigger.

Your Body Changes

Engagement or lightening, the process of the baby 'dropping' down into the pelvic cavity in preparation for delivery, may occur any time now. In some women (particularly those who have given birth before), it may not happen until labour starts.

Your cervix is ripening (softening) in preparation for baby's passage. As it effaces (thins) and dilates (opens), the soft plug of mucus keeping it sealed tight may be dislodged. This mass, which has the appealing name of mucus plug, may be tinged red or pink, and is also referred to as the equally explicit 'show'.

A pregnancy is considered full-term from 37 to 42 weeks. Only 5 per cent of expectant women actually give birth on their estimated date of delivery, and first-time mums are more likely to go past their due date. If you've delivered a baby before, however, you are more likely to give birth within four days of your EDD.

What You Feel Like

If the baby has dropped, you may be running to the toilet more than ever. He also may be sending shockwaves through your pelvis as he settles further down onto the pelvic floor. On the upside, you can finally breathe as he pulls away from your lungs and diaphragm. Braxton-Hicks contractions may be more frequent this month as you draw nearer to delivery. You're close enough to be on the lookout for the real thing, however. How will you recognize them?

Real contractions will:

· Be felt in the back and possibly radiate around to the abdomen.
· *Not* subside when you move around or change positions.
· Increase in intensity as time passes.
· Come at roughly regular intervals (early on, this may be from 20 to 45 minutes apart).
· Increase in intensity with activities such as walking.

Other signs that labour is on its way include amniotic fluid leaks in either a gush or a trickle (your 'waters breaking'), sudden diarrhoea and the appearance of the mucus plug. Keep in mind, however, that for many women, the waters do not break until active labour sets in.

At the Doctor

Unless you are scheduled for a planned Caesarean, your doctor will probably perform an internal examination with each visit to check your cervix for changes that indicate approaching labour.

Checking Your Cervix

Your provider will be checking your cervix for signs that it is preparing for your baby's passage. She'll also be taking note of any descent or dropping of the baby toward the pelvis, called the station. Take the numbers you hear with a grain of salt, however. Although you may start effacing and dilating now, it's still anyone's guess as to when labour will begin, and it could be a few more weeks yet.

On Your Mind

You're likely tired but happy as you pack and prepare for the big day. Just remember the 'estimated' bit in 'estimated delivery date' to avoid a big letdown if baby is tardy.

Tired of Being Pregnant

You are *so* ready to have this baby. Nothing fits, not even your shoes. You can't sleep for more than a few hours at a time. Your belly itches and your breasts ache. You look toward your due date like a long distance runner approaching the end of a marathon. As you waddle towards the finish line, enjoy these final sensations of your child moving inside you – the funny little hiccups, the elbow and knee bumps parading across your belly, and the subtle nudges that remind you you're not alone even when no one else is around.

When your cervix hasn't budged and your due date has come and gone, you may be tempted to try one of those surefire homemade labour inducers that every pregnant woman hears about. Castor oil, herbal concoctions, spicy food and sex are just a few methods bandied about in pregnancy chat rooms everywhere. Unfortunately, some may only succeed in making you nauseous, while others may pose a real danger. Even if you're embarrassed, you need to check with your doctor or midwife before taking matters into your own hands. A good health-care provider will listen and won't laugh, letting you know what's safe and what isn't.

Irritable and Anxious

As sleep gets more and more elusive and your discomfort level goes up and up, you may find yourself easily provoked. The best short-term solution to keeping your cool? Stay clear of encounters with people you just know will irritate you (whether they mean to or not), and ask your partner to be the front person on all 'Anything yet?' questions.

First-time mums may find themselves overwhelmed with anxiety now that birth is so near. Take a deep breath, go over what you learned in childbirth class (repeatedly, if this helps to ease your mind), and talk with your partner or labour coach about ways to relax and get past the anxious feelings. It's perfectly natural to be fearful of the unknown, but don't let fear wrest control of your labour from you.

Even if you have been through pregnancy already, you may still be anxious about baby's arrival. Perhaps you're following a different kind of labour and birth plan, or you're concerned about how your other child will react to his new brother or sister. Again, talk it out with your partner, ask your provider any questions that may still be on your mind about labour and delivery, and remember that you've been through this once and you'll make it through again.

Excited and Happy

How could you not be excited? You're finally going to meet the little one you've known only through kicks, hiccups and grainy ultrasound images. Will she look like you? What will you do when you get to hold her for the first time? Relish these final days of exhilaration and anticipation – they are truly unique.

Gearing Up for the Big Event

Since baby's timetable is somewhat unpredictable, start getting your affairs in order at the beginning of this month. Cover all personal, professional and family bases to ensure a smooth transition from home to hospital and back home again.

Finalize the Birth Plan

Double-check with your doctor that a copy of your birth plan has been put into your chart, and verify any changes you might have made to the plan since your first review together. Provide your labour coach with an extra copy just in case the original is misplaced.

Pack Your Bag

You'll probably pack and unpack your bag a half dozen times this month, making sure you have everything you could possibly need. Don't go crazy with books, notebook computersor other work or entertainment equipment. You'll be too busy with labour, delivery and the blissful preoccupation of meeting and caring for your child.

Essentials you should have:

- **Pain-relief tools for labour.** Things like massage balls, a picture for focusing on through contractions, a water bottle and so on.
- **Music to labour by.** Check with your hospital or birth centre in advance, to see if a small portable stereo is acceptable. If not, you can always bring personal headphones.
- **Snacks.** Make sure it's something that won't turn your stomach if you see or smell it during labour.
- **A camera.** For capturing baby's arrival (or the moments shortly thereafter). Don't forget the batteries and film (or an extra memory card)!
- **Stopwatch, clock or watch with a second hand.** For timing contractions.
- **Several nightgowns.** With button or snap fronts if you're going to nurse.
- **Extra underwear.** Make this comfortable but not your best – it'll probably end up with some postpartum bloodstains.
- **Sanitary pads.** The hospital will provide you with some, but extras are good to have on hand.
- **Phone numbers.** Make sure your partner has names and numbers of the people you'll want to clue in immediately on the new arrival.
- **A small gift from baby to any siblings.** A 'Hello big sister/brother'

gift can make the introduction smoother.

- **A picture of the kids.** Taping a picture of big brother or sister to your newborn's crib is a good way to emphasize your first child's important new role in the family.
- **Glasses or contact lenses.** Make sure you can see the baby after he's finally here.
- **Warm socks and/or slippers.** Those hospital floors can be cold.
- **A dressing gown.** For hallway walks to the nursery.
- **A baby blanket.** For baby's return home. Let your partner bring the car seat on discharge day so you aren't overwhelmed with luggage.
- **Toiletries.** Toothbrush, toothpaste and other basics.
- **Shower supplies.** You'll be given an opportunity to shower at the hospital, so pack shampoo and other necessities.
- **A going-home outfit for both you and baby.** Pack a set of newborn clothes, and make sure you bring something loose and comfortable to wear yourself.

If you're breast-feeding, you might also pack:

- **Nursing bras.** If you don't have any yet, a bra with a front fastener will work well as a stand-in for now.
- **A box of nursing pads.** For when your milk comes in.
- **Vitamin E oil or lanolin ointment.** For sore or cracked nipples.

Don't put your pre-pregnancy jeans in your hospital bag. You're sure to be sorely disappointed. While you'll lose a large percentage of the weight you've gained this past nine months, it will take some time to return to your old shape and size. If the thought of putting on maternity clothes yet again postpartum is too depressing, buy a comfortable but stretchy 'coming-home' outfit in a new-mum-friendly size. Remember that trousers or jeans can rub against stitches!

Recruit Help Now!

Now is the time to take up friends, family and neighbours on their offers of assistance.

If they ask if they can help, by all means take them up on it. Make a list and schedule assignments. Give friends that are good in the kitchen cooking requests, so you can have a supply of frozen, home-cooked meals on hand for easy dinners. If you have other children, charge your husband or partner with making sure their school, extracurricular and social schedules are covered.

Feel like you need some live-in help to get you through the first week or so? Ask a mummy-expert, maybe even your own mum, to come for a visit. Sound out the idea with your mate; he may feel this is a special 'just the three of you' family time, but also might reconsider if he hears your reasons. Just make sure your guest isn't someone who will be driving you bonkers after a couple of days.

Having a Caesarean section? You'll be recovering from major surgery as well as going through all those new-mum adjustments. It's essential you have adequate rest and support so you can heal and care for your new baby. It may be tempting to leave hospital as soon as possible to start family life in earnest, especially if you have older children, but don't fall into the trap of resuming all your normal tasks too soon. Get as much rest as you can and avoid lifting or driving for six weeks after the birth.

Finalize Maternity Leave Plans

If you're working right up until your due date, start clearing the decks early in the month. Make sure colleagues and managers are regularly apprised of where outstanding projects stand, and try to treat every day as if it may be your last before leave. The more you enable things to flow smoothly in your absence, the less likely you are to get calls at home.

Talk to your supervisor about communication in your absence. If you want to remain incommunicado (and you have every right to do so), make your feelings known. You might think about setting a limit on any contact you do agree to, such as e-mails only, which may be easier to answer at your leisure when baby is asleep, or phone calls only in a certain window of time each day. Be sure to outline circumstances that you would consider important enough to be disturbed for. Remember – this is your time off to both recuperate and get to know your child. Your workplace will survive. For more on working through pregnancy, see Chapter 9.

Hurry Up and Wait (When Baby Is Late)

You've finally reached that magic EDD number and... nothing. No fanfare, no contractions and definitely no baby. Disappointed, you resign yourself to yet another day of pregnancy. Don't be too depressed. Instead, try to stay busy and if you feel up to it, get out and about. A nice long walk may be just what your little one needs for inspiration. Sitting at home, analyzing every twitch of your abdomen and watching the hours crawl by will only make the waiting longer.

I'm 1 week overdue. Will my doctor induce me if I request it?
Whether or not to induce depends on a number of factors. Is the cervix effaced or dilated? Are you fairly sure your due date was accurate to begin with? Have you had a previous Caesarean? Generally speaking, if you've hit the 42-week mark, you have no history of Caesarean and your provider thinks induction is indicated, she will schedule one for you. For more on induction, turn to Chapter 18.

Unless you have a precise 28-day cycle and are positive of the exact day that sperm met egg, gestational dating can be fuzzy at best. If you are one week or more past the EDD, your provider will order additional tests, including a biophysical profile, which includes a non-stress test (NST) and ultrasound assessment of amniotic fluid levels and foetal size. These tools give a much better picture of whether or not baby is ready to arrive.

Babies who stay in the womb for 42 weeks or longer are considered post-term or postdate. Postdate pregnancies may develop macrosomia, or large body size of 4,000grams (8lb 13oz) or more that may make it difficult to pass through the birth canal. A postdate foetus may also pass meconium, the black tarry stool that is baby's first bowel movement. If meconium is released into the amniotic fluid, it has the potential to cause foetal distress by blocking the airway. That's why regular assessment of a post-date pregnancy is extremely important.

Just for Dads

It's showtime! Finally, you'll be able to get into the parenting act on a more hands-on level. As the baby's due date approaches, remember that your partner needs you more than ever. Spoil her a little – or even a lot.

Getting Her to the Hospital

Having nightmares about having to deliver the baby in the back seat of your Ford Mondeo? Perhaps it will ease your mind to hear that the average first-time mum is in labour for about 14 hours (women in later pregnancies tend to have shorter labours – around an 8-hour average), more than enough time to get to the hospital.

Remembering everything in the thrill of the big moment may be hard, so make yourself a checklist and keep it on your dash: one overnight bag, your list of phone numbers, plenty of change for phone calls or a fully charged mobile phone, and of course, one labouring mum-to-be. And make a habit of filling the car's fuel tank every time it reaches the half-empty mark so you won't have to stop for petrol.

Bring your credit card or a pocketful of change for your long list of phone calls. Many hospitals do not allow mobile phone use inside the building, due to the risk of interference with sensitive medical equipment. Labour takes a long time, so bring a snack.

False Alarms

Many women hit the hospital certain that they're just hours away from birth, only to be told they're just a few centimetres dilated. There is no bigger letdown for a very pregnant woman, particularly one who is past her due date, to be sent home from the hospital with baby still on board. She may get tearful, frustrated, exasperated and convinced that she'll be pregnant forever. Even though you may be disappointed by the delay as well, give her a good shoulder to cry on and offer some extra TLC.

Taking the Strains

Taking over phone duty this month can help ease your partner's stress significantly. The chances are that family, friends, neighbours and anyone else who knows the big day is approaching will be calling for a status report. As the due date draws near, this can be a nuisance, but when the date has come and gone, it escalates into the unbearable zone. Let your partner know you'll field the phone calls for now and pass along anything of consequence. If it gets to be too much of a deluge, you might gently remind your callers that they're on your list to be contacted once something does occur.

Chapter 18

Labour and Delivery

Even if you've read just about everything about labour and delivery, taken copious notes in childbirth class and questioned all your friends on their experiences, you'll still find your labour experiences different in some way from the others. Every woman's labour is unique, and so comparisons of length, progress and pain perception can be inaccurate, or even discouraging. Follow your own path, and you'll do fine.

Get Ready: Baby and Your Body in Labour

Labour is hard work (don't let anyone tell you otherwise), but it's also the most rewarding work you'll ever do.

Contractions

The first signal of labour is contractions – the tightening and release of your uterus that helps propel your baby down the birth canal. These contractions are different than the Braxton-Hicks you may have had, in that they occur at regular intervals, are painful, and are slowly but surely opening the door (i.e. cervix) for baby's exit.

You don't need to rush to the hospital after your first contraction. But you should call your doctor or midwife and let them know that labour has started and how far apart contractions are (from the beginning of one to the start of the next). Your doctor will let you know at what point you should head for the hospital or birth centre. Until then, you can labour in the comfort and privacy of your own home. However, if the pain starts to be more than you can handle without professional help, call your doctor again and bring her up to date with the situation. Below are some early pain-relief options you can try at home.

Preparation

When you arrive at your birth centre or hospital, the nursing staff will prep, or prepare. you for labour and delivery. What prepping involves depends on facility policy and doctor preference, but here are some procedures you may encounter.

Suit Up

You'll change into your hospital gown or gear from home. Try not to wear a lot of jewellery or other extraneous items that may get lost.

Baby Monitor

The chances are that you've experienced the foetal monitor during a visit to your doctor, so this part of the procedure may be familiar to you. The monitor will give you a look at your contractions, and it will allow you and your coach to see when one is coming and, more importantly, when it seems to be almost over. It will also pick up foetal heart sounds and alert you to any stress the baby may be experiencing from oxygen deprivation or problems with the umbilical cord. An internal monitor may be used if you are considered to be at high risk. For legal reasons you will be monitored for 20 minutes when you arrive, but if there are no concerns, you should be able to move about after this. For more on foetal monitoring, see Chapter 5.

tips

If you don't want to be chained to your bed during labor, find out if your birth facility has foetal monitors that use telemetry technology. These wireless monitors strap on like a regular external device, but you don't have to remain plugged into anything. You may have to remain in the same room with the base unit, however, depending on the type of system. There are even telemetry units that are waterproof in case a mum wants to ease labour pains with hydrotherapy.

Get Set: Pain-Relief Options

In early labour, when contractions are getting intense but are still not close enough so that you should leave for the hospital, there are a few ways you can ease the pain.

Non-medical Solutions

First, have plenty of pillows on hand. Experiment with different positions, such as on all fours, against a wall and leaning against someone or something while bent forward at the waist.

Back labour, which occurs when baby's face is toward your abdomen rather than your spine, can cause severe lower back pain. Ask your partner to try massage or a warm water bottle to ease contractions. The soothing jets of a whirlpool tub can do wonders if you have one. However, if your waters have broken, check with your care provider.

Keep positive, supportive people around you. Let your partner be your buffer, and clear out any distractions. Try to remain focused on riding through and past the contraction. Fix your eyes on something that relaxes you and practise the breathing exercises you learned in childbirth class to keep the oxygen and blood flowing. Don't hyperventilate. Talk or groan through the height of the contraction if it helps.

It's difficult to remember to relax when you're in the middle of a really big, really uncomfortable contraction. However, letting go in between contractions can help ease your mind and body and loosen you up for impending delivery. You may have learned a few relaxation exercises in childbirth class. If so, now is the time to try them, as they can make the pain more manageable.

Progressive relaxation, which is a series of muscle tightening and release, is a good way to release your stress. Make sure you're in comfortable clothes in a soothing atmosphere (i.e. quiet and perhaps dimly lit). Recline with your head and back elevated, and start tensing and then releasing each muscle group, from your head to your toes. Breathe in with the tension, and blow it out with the release. Try to clear your head of everything but the sensation at hand. If you practise this prior to labour, it can be a good tool for managing some of the early pain, when contractions are still relatively far apart.

TENS Machines

Transcutaneous Electrical Nerve Stimulation (TENS) is an increasingly popular form of pain relief. This small battery-operated machine is attached to your body with adhesive pads (rather like those body-toning devices). A small electrical current is passed through your skin, reducing the pain messages being sent to your brain and stimulating feel-good endorphins. This is a non-invasive form of pain relief that can be used with any other method except in water, and you are free to move about while using it. You also have the advantage that you are in charge of the dial – it can feel good to be in charge of something during labour. Some hospitals do have TENS machines, but to be sure of having one many women opt to hire one privately.

Pharmaceutical Options

Once you arrive at the hospital, you will have analgesics and anaesthetics available for pain relief if you choose to have them.

Analgesics

Analgesics deaden pain by depressing your nervous system. They make you sleepy and help you rest between contractions. Although some of these drugs, such as Pethedine, may allow you to nap between contractions, you remain conscious (if a bit giddy) under their influence.

Pain relief in labour was roundly condemned for many centuries, partly on biblical grounds (think Eve and the apple), until Queen Victoria requested and was administered chloroform for the birth of her eighth and ninth children. The births of both Prince Leopold and Princess Beatrice were attended by D. John Snow, a pioneer in anaesthetic use. After Prince Leopold was born in 1853, the Queen praised the relief chloroform provided, thus legitimizing the obstetrical use of anaesthetic and the further advancement of the field.

General Anaesthesia

Less commonly, you may also receive either a general or local (regional) anaesthetic. A general anaesthetic brings about a complete loss of consciousness, or 'puts you to sleep'. General anaesthesia is usually only used in cases of an emergency Caesarean section where there isn't adequate time to prep the patient with a local anaesthetic. Newborns arriving under the influence of a general anaesthetic may be drowsy and slow to respond due to the effects of the anaesthesia.

Local Anaesthesia

Local anaesthesia, also called regional anaesthesia, numbs only a specific portion of the body and leaves you awake and alert. The most commonly used local anaesthesia is probably the lumbar epidural. Injected into the space between two vertebrae of your lower back (the epidural space), this type of anaesthesia is administered when you are well into labour, and will temporarily numb the nerves all the way from your belly button to your knees. An epidural takes 20 minutes to start working and can also lower your blood pressure. For this reason, you'll be put on the foetal monitor and hooked up to an IV fluid drip if you're given an epidural.

Some providers may require you to wait until you reach a certain dilation benchmark or stage of labour to have an epidural, but if you are being induced, an epidural may be in order earlier, since you may experience a lot of pain before there is any major progress in the dilation of your cervix. Most doctors will give you more time to push with an epidural because your sensation is impaired. If you have concerns about epidural timing, discuss them with your health-care provider.

The epidural is administered through a small plastic catheter in your back. An anaesthesiologist will place the epidural catheter and administer the local anaesthetic agent. Before he starts, your lower back will be draped and the insertion spot swabbed with antiseptic or iodine. You may be asked to pull your knees and chin toward your chest so your spine is more visible. The catheter is inserted in the space between the fourth and fifth vertebrae, and the anaesthesia is injected into it. You may feel a slight stinging sensation down your legs, but your breathing and the involuntary muscles working those contractions won't be affected. The insertion of an epidural catheter allows anaesthetics to be administered on an as-needed basis, and is useful should a Caesarean ultimately be required.

After insertion, the doctor will secure the catheter and you can get comfortable again. Watch the foetal monitor for the start of the next contraction. You'll be amazed at how what was turning you inside out a moment ago is barely perceptible now. The numbness will take several hours to wear off and may restrict your movements during the birth, but an epidural can be a great pain-management tool.

A spinal block, like an epidural, is administered in the lower back. However, a spinal is delivered directly into the fluid around your spinal cord, not into the spaces between your vertebrae, as with an epidural. Used right at delivery only, or during a Caesarean, the spinal block will numb you all the way down from your ribcage.

Women who would like to have the pain relief benefits of an epidural but would also like to retain the ability to move around during labour may be candidates for a low-dose combination spinal epidural, sometimes referred to as a walking epidural. An epidural catheter is inserted, and an injection of a narcotic is administered into the spinal fluid by using a smaller needle that fits through the epidural catheter. A walking epidural is usually faster-acting than a conventional epidural, and it allows you to retain enough sensation to move and walk, which can speed the labour process.

Other anaesthetic blocks that are used less frequently include:

·   A caudal block is administered into the bony area right at the end of your spine, and affects the abdominal and pelvic muscles.
·   A saddle block is a type of low spinal that numbs a more limited area of your body – your perineum, inner thighs and bottom.
·   With a paracervical block, the anaesthetic is injected into either side of your cervix during labour to numb the area.
·   With a pudendal block, the anaesthetic is administered to the nerves around the vagina and pelvic floor to help control pain when the baby's head bulges into your cervix.

Go! Labour in Three Acts

Labour is a series of three distinct stages, aptly called first, second and third stages. For most women, the longest distance to cover is the first stage, which lasts from the earliest signs of labour right through baby's descent into the birth canal in preparation for stage two – pushing. Stage three consists of delivering the placenta, which some mothers feel is a piece of cake after all the hard work involved in baby's arrival.

First Stage

The first stage of labour is actually a three-part act itself, consisting of early (latent), active and transition (descent) labour.

During the early phase, the cervix effaces (thins) and dilates (opens). This ripening process may have started several weeks ago, well before the regular contractions of early labour began (see Chapter 17). Now, your cervix will dilate to about 4–5cm (1³/₈–2in). Contractions will arrive every 15–20 minutes and last 60–90 seconds. If your partner or coach isn't around, now is the time to contact him so he can be by your side. Then get in touch with your doctor or midwife, who will tell you at what point you should head to the hospital or birth facility.

Try to stay up and moving through contractions as much as you can, to let gravity help your baby descend. Consider a light liquid snack (e.g. broth or juice) to charge your energy reserves for the long road ahead. Rest if possible. Try the breathing and relaxation techniques you picked up in childbirth class, and coach-assisted massage or showering to get you through these first few hours. Then leave for the hospital and the next stage – active labour.

> It can be tempting to dash off to the hospital at the first twinge of labour, but remember that birth is usually a long process — particularly if this is your first baby. You will be more relaxed in your own environment while you can still stand the pain without too much trouble, and it can be very disheartening to hurtle off to the maternity unit just to be told you are only 2cm (³/₄in) dilated.

In active labour, your contractions are coming closer together regularly, perhaps 3–5 minutes apart, and they can be intense, lasting 45 seconds. These strong contractions are dilating your cervix from about 4–5cm (1³/₈–2in) to around 8cm (3¹/₈in), when transition begins.

Once you reach the birth centre or hospital, you'll be quickly prepped as described earlier and given an internal exam to check the progress of your cervix. The baby's position will be checked, and you will probably be hooked up to a foetal monitor to assess the baby's well-being. (See Chapter 5 for more on foetal monitoring.)

Other signs that active labour is in progress:

· Your membranes rupture. If the amniotic sac hasn't already broken, it will now or very soon.

- You bleed from your vagina. More of the mucus plug is being expelled.
- You need air. Put those cleansing breaths and other breathing techniques into practice. Your hardworking uterus needs oxygen.
- Your back *really* hurts. The baby's head is pushing on your backbone. Massage may help.
- You have muscle cramp. Again, massage may help the ill-timed spasms.
- You're exhausted and physically spent. Remember what you're working toward. Let your partner know how you're feeling so he can help you and get you whatever he can to keep moving forward.

Don't feel inadequate or guilty about asking for pain medication at any point if you want and need it. You wouldn't hesitate to take novocaine if you were having a wisdom tooth pulled, yet having a 3.6kg (8oz) child pulled through a 10cm (4in) opening doesn't qualify? Pain medication is a tool, just like your breathing exercises. Wisely used, it can result in a better birth experience for both you and your child.

Once your cervix reaches 8cm ($3^1/8$in) and contractions start coming one on top of another to get you to full dilation, transition has arrived. Because of the frequency of contractions and the overwhelming urge to push, this is the most difficult part of labour. Fortunately, it culminates in your child's delivery once you bridge those final 2cm ($^3/4$in) to being fully dilated.

During transition:

- You could be nauseous and may even vomit.
- You have chills or sweats, and your muscles twitch.
- Your back *really, really* hurts.
- Contractions are just minutes apart, if even that.
- There is pressure in your rectum from the baby.
- You are absolutely exhausted.
- You may feel like pushing even though your cervix is not yet fully dilated.

Although every fibre of your body may be screaming 'PUSH!', you need to hold back just a few moments more. Your cervix is almost, but not quite, open far enough for baby's safe passage. Take quick shallow breaths and resist the urge until your doctor or midwife gives you the go-ahead to push.

Second Stage, or PUSH!

Your cervix has made it to 10cm (4in), and you are finally allowed to push. This second stage can last anywhere from a few minutes (with second or subsequent babies) to several hours. Your contractions will still arrive regularly, but they aren't quite as close together, a welcome relief. Pushing is very hard work, but the sensations may change from the intense gripping you've experienced to more of a stinging or burning sensation.

If possible, try to find a pushing position that doesn't attempt to defy gravity. Instead, use gravity to your advantage by kneeling, squatting, or sitting up with your legs and knees spread far apart. Stirrups may be available, but don't feel forced into using them if they don't work for you.

Your birth attendant and/or coach will let you know when the peak of the contraction occurs, the optimum time for pushing effectively. Use whatever it takes to push effectively. If that means moaning, grunting and other primal sounds that make your prenatal snoring sound like a lullaby in comparison, go for it. The people attending your birth have probably seen just about everything. Don't be embarrassed, because it won't even phase them.

The emergence of the head at your vaginal opening starts with a small patch of skin visible during the peak of a push. The patch may recede when you rest, but will reappear at the next contraction. Unless your baby is arriving in a breech position, the head will finally crown, or bulge out of your vaginal opening. You may be asked to stop pushing momentarily, as the baby's head is ready to emerge, in order to prevent perineal tearing. Panting can help you suppress the urge. The obstetrician or midwife may decide on an episiotomy if your skin doesn't appear to be willing to stretch another millimetre, or they may attempt perineal massage.

Finally, the head slides face down past the perineum and is eased out carefully by the birth attendant to prevent injury to the baby. The attendant may wipe the eyes, nose and mouth, and suction any mucus or fluid from her upper respiratory tract. It's all downhill from here as the rest of the body slides out.

As your baby leaves the quiet, dim warmth of the womb for the bright lights and big noises of the outside world, his respiratory reflexes kick in and the newborn lungs fill with air for the first time. He'll probably test out those lungs with a full-fledged wail.

Your doctor will place the baby on your stomach for introductions, usually with the umbilical cord still attached.

The cord will continue to pulse with blood flow for a few minutes. The timing of the actual clamping and severing of the cord will depend upon your doctor or midwife, and this is a matter of some debate in childbirth circles. Some professionals believe that waiting until pulsation has stopped, or even until after the placenta is delivered, improves baby's circulation and blood pressure and reduces mum's chance of haemorrhaging. Other professionals cite a higher incidence of jaundice in newborns with delayed cord cuts, and believe in clamping and cutting earlier. You may want to talk it over with your doctor if you have concerns about the timing of the cord cut. If baby requires resuscitation because the cord is tightly wrapped around a body part, or if the cord is exceedingly short, it will be cut sooner.

Most doctors will give dad, or even mum, the option of cutting the cord in an uncomplicated birth. Don't feel bad if it isn't your cup of tea, especially if either one of you is a bit squeamish. Better to spend the time cuddling your baby than being picked up off the delivery room floor.

What is umbilical cord banking?
The umbilical cord blood contains stem cells, from which all organs and tissues are built. Cord blood collected immediately after birth is placed in a collection kit and flown to a facility where it is cryogenically frozen and 'banked' for later use if needed. The theory behind cord banking is that if your child ever develops a disease or condition requiring stem-cell treatment, the cord blood can be thawed and used for her treatment. If it matches certain biological markers, cord blood can be used to treat other family members as well. However, banking is cost-prohibitive for many and requires an annual storage fee for as long as you'd like to keep the cord blood frozen.

Third, or, You Aren't Done Yet

The third stage of labour is the delivery of the placenta. The entire placenta must be expelled to prevent bleeding complications later on. Contractions will continue, and your doctor may press down on your abdomen and massage your uterus, or tug gently on the end of the umbilical cord hanging from your vagina. You may also be injected with the hormone Pitocin (oxytocin) to step up your contractions and expel the placenta. You'll be given pushing directives again, but this part will seem like a piece of cake, given the task you've just completed.

Once the placenta is out, any stitches you require to repair tearing or episiotomy incisions will be put in. A local anaesthetic will be injected to deaden the area if you aren't still anaesthetized from an epidural.

Caesarean Section

A Caesarean birth may be scheduled for you if you have a breech baby or other complications or conditions that indicate the need for a Caesarean. It may also be performed in emergency situations where the foetus is in distress. A Caesarean is major abdominal surgery that carries with it all the risks of infection and complication that any surgical procedure does.

On the positive side, with a planned Caesarean your due date is your due date, and no contractions are necessary unless you begin to go into labour before the date.

In Advance of the Surgery

If you have any advance warning about your Caesarean, you'll probably be offered an epidural or spinal rather than general anaesthesia. Before the procedure begins, you'll be prepped. A nurse will shave the area of the incision, and your arm will be hooked up to an intravenous line to receive fluids as well as pain medication. You may also be asked to drink an antacid solution called sodium citrate to neutralize your stomach acid.

Before the procedure begins you will have a catheter inserted into your bladder. The anesthetic block will give you little control over the muscles that control urine flow, so the catheter will do the work for you both during and after the procedure. Catheter insertion can be uncomfortable, so ask that it be inserted after you've received your anaesthetic block (which probably likely be in the operating room).

In the Operating Room

Once you're prepared, you will be wheeled to the operating room. In the operating room, the anaesthetist will get you to roll on your side and pull your knees toward your chest, or sit with your legs dangling off the table, while he inserts a fine needle and catheter for an epidural or spinal block into your back. You'll then be asked to lie flat on your back with your arms straight out to the sides. A curtain just a few feet high will be positioned at your chest to keep the surgical field (the area where all the action is) sterile. This will also block your view of the procedure, so if you're determined to see baby the moment she emerges, you will need to ask for an appropriately placed mirror as early as possible.

A severe headache known as postdural or post-puncture spinal headache is an uncommon but highly uncomfortable potential side effect of spinal blocks and epidurals. It is caused by the change in spinal fluid pressure that occurs if spinal fluid leaks out into the epidural space during or after the procedure. It may be more common in spinal blocks because of the larger needle size used. Rest and fluids usually resolve the problem, but in some cases an injection of blood into the epidural space, called a blood patch, may be required to seal the puncture site.

The obstetrician will make an incision, and the baby's head, perfectly round because she hasn't done battle with the birth canal, will be lifted out first and her mouth and nose will be suctioned. As your doctor helps your baby out of the incision, you'll feel a strange pulling sensation. Once the cord is cut you'll be able to finally see your baby, although perhaps briefly, before she is taken for assessment and a quick clean-up by the nursing staff. Your incision will be stitched closed, and you'll be wheeled off to the recovery room, where your little one will meet up with you once again. The entire surgical procedure will only take about 30 –45 minutes.

Emergency Caesarean

If your Caesarean is performed under emergency circumstances, things could move quickly and you'll have fewer options. You may also be given a general anaesthetic that will make you unconscious. Most dads are asked to step outside when general anaesthesia has been administered, but you can talk to your doctor about special circumstances during childbirth.

Induction

In cases where you are definitely 41 weeks or further along and it seems as if your child has decided she is perfectly content with spending her infancy in your womb, your doctor may recommend induction. Inducing labour involves both helping the cervix ripen for baby's passage and stimulating uterine contractions. Both are important for a successful labour and delivery; if the cervix is not adequately effaced and dilated the chance of interventions (e.g. Caesarean or use of forceps) increases.

Your doctor may use one of several methods to facilitate cervical ripening, including membrane stripping and amniotomy (manual breaking of the membranes or 'bag of waters'). Stripping, or sweeping, of the membranes is simply the separation of the amniotic membrane from the wall of the cervix. Your provider will insert her finger in the cervix and gently sweep it between the amniotic membrane and the uterine wall.

If she opts for amniotomy, she'll use an instrument with a small blunt hook on the end (an amnihook) to break through the amniotic sac. If labour does not start on its own within 24 hours, scheduled induction may be necessary because of the risk of infection for the baby.

Because a scheduled induction is more successful when the cervix is prepared for the experience, your practitioner may recommend an application of prostaglandin gel to your cervix the day before. The prostaglandin helps to ripen the cervix for labour and delivery. In some cases, it may be used alone as an inducing agent. The gel is applied to your vagina with a swab, while the baby's heart rate is assessed with a foetal monitor. More than one application may be ordered.

fact

A study published in the journal *Obstetrics & Gynecology* in 2002 found that the rate of labor induction in the United States more than doubled between 1989 and 1998. And according to the US Centers for Disease Control ,more than one in five births were induced in 2001. Researchers attribute the increase to earlier prenatal care, wider availability of induction agents, and non-medical reasons such as convenience for the patient or doctor. Because induction can cause intense contractions and result in a longer labour, its use should always be carefully considered.

Pitocin – a synthetic formulation of the hormone oxytocin that stimulates uterine contractions – may be prescribed as an inducing agent. The hormone is given intravenously, and you will be hooked up to a foetal monitor to monitor your baby's progress.

After Birth

The pinnacle of nine months of physical chaos and emotional oscillation, of queasy stomachs, lost car keys, aches, pains and hair-trigger laughter and tears, has arrived. Your baby is here, placed skin to skin to feel her mother's outside warmth for the very first time.

Meeting Baby

A thousand different feelings and emotions, from utter exhaustion to indescribable joy, will flood you as you look down at that little scrunched face, still adjusting to its new waterless environment. Wrapped in a blanket to keep her warm, she looks so perfect yet so vulnerable.

If you're planning to breast-feed, you can nurse her while you get acquainted, or even in the recovery room if you've had a Caesarean. It's awe-inspiring how she knows just what to do, instinctively rooting for your breast with her eyes barely open, and then latching on. Spend as long as you want getting familiar and let baby's daddy share in the bonding, too. This is a precious time for your new family.

Baby's First 'Doctor's Visit'

After you've met your child, he'll need some initial tests and treatments to ensure a healthy welcome into the world. The first is an Apgar test, which is simply an assessment of baby's reactivity, health and appearance at birth. Created by noted pediatrician Dr Virginia Apgar, the Apgar measures Appearance (skin colour), Pulse, Grimace (reflexes), Activity and Respiration. The Apgar is given just one minute after birth, and again five minutes after that. The attendant will assign a score of 0–2 for each category and add them together for the total Apgar. An average score is 7–10.

After the Apgar, your newborn will be measured and weighed, and have prints taken of his feet and fingers. Silver nitrate or antibiotic eyedrops or ointment may be put in his eyes to prevent infection from anything he encountered in the birth canal. He'll also receive a vitamin K injection to prevent bleeding problems; a heelstick blood draw to test for PKU and hypothyroidism; and in some hospitals a hepatitis B vaccine. Further tests may be administered if you have a chronic illness or experienced complications during pregnancy. If you have diabetes, for example, your newborn will have his blood glucose (sugar) levels tested.

Taking Care of Mum

After the birth, you'll have some assistance cleaning up and will be given a good supply of superabsorbent sanitary pads. You'll also be provided with a peribottle, a plastic squirt bottle used to cleanse and soothe your perineal area with warm water each time you use the toilet.

You'll be expelling lochia for up to six weeks following birth, whether you've had a vaginal birth or a Caesarean. Lochia – a mixture of blood, mucus and tissue that comes from the site of implantation of the placenta – will be quite heavy in the days immediately following the birth, so don't be alarmed.

If bleeding is soaking through more than a pad per hour, let your doctor, midwife, or nurse know. This could be a sign that a piece of placenta is still retained in your uterus.

If you've had a Caesarean, you'll spend some time in the recovery area before heading to your hospital room. Your incision will be checked regularly, and pain medication will be administered as needed. The next day, you'll be encouraged to walk as soon as possible to get your digestive tract active again, and you'll be asked about your wind and toilet habits ad nauseum. The nursing staff is just trying to ensure everything is returning to normal in gastrointestinal land.

Hospital Stay

In general, your baby can sleep in your hospital room with you and you can begin the process of learning to care and comfort him. It's a marvellous way to promote early bonding. However, if you are exhausted and your little guy seems to be having a problem getting to sleep, don't hesitate to get some help from the nursing staff.

If you need a nap, they can wheel him down to the nursery for a few hours while you sleep. Childbirth, whether vaginally or by Caesarean, takes a physical toll that you need to recover from in order to be anythign like an effective parent.

For the same reason, don't feel bad about keeping visitors to a minimum. Your hospital will have a visitor's policy, which will help somewhat. While introducing immediate family to their new relative is important, friends, neighbours and colleagues can wait. At many facilities, you can also request that the switchboard hold phone calls to your room. Anyone who has a cold or other infection, even a family member, should not come in contact with your baby now because of the risk of infection, and hand-washing is a must for all visitors. Her little immune system is just starting to rev up.

For more on introducing siblings to their new brother or sister, see Chapter 11.

Recovery from a Caesarean will take a bit longer than from a vaginal delivery. When you laugh, sneeze or cough, hold onto your incision with both hands. Using extra pillows for support over the incision area will allow you to cuddle and breast-feed your baby in comfort.

If you are planning to breast-feed, now is the perfect time to get your technique down. Your nurses will likely ask you how breast-feeding is progressing, and they may request you to write down the time and frequency of nursing so they can assess baby's progress. They can also examine your latching technique to help you troubleshoot if things aren't yet going smoothly. In some cases, there may even be a lactation consultant available, and hospitals frequently offer breast-feeding classes to their new mother inpatients. For more on breast-feeding, see Chapter 19.

Remember that while it will take a few days for your breasts to start manufacturing milk, you are still providing your child with nutrient-rich colostrum, the prelude to breast milk. When your milk does arrive (or 'come in'), about the third day after delivery, your breasts may be quite swollen, hard and sore. This engorgement will be relieved upon nursing. If you're going the bottle route, cold packs and supportive bras or binding can ease the discomfort.

The tenderness of engorgement usually passes in two to three days, and may be relieved by mild analgesics as prescribed by your doctor. While you wait for your milk supply to dry up again (usually a period of about two weeks), you can use nursing pads to prevent leaks.

On Your Mind

Mortified by the possibility of losing control – both physically and emotionally – during labour? Childbirth is hard, painful work, and you need to work through it in your own way. The people around you are medical professionals and know this. Pain, and the ultimate goal of meeting your child, is a great motivator for getting past feelings of fear or bashfulness.

Many women who were once shy or self-conscious about their body find that pregnancy and motherhood pretty much eradicate any lingering traces of modesty they may have once had. When you're in labour you don't care if the attending doctor is animal, vegetable or mineral; your mind and body are entirely focused on the impending arrival of your child. After they've been through the birth experience, many women find that there's virtually nothing that can embarrass them.

Just for Dads

Until today, your most important function may have seemed to be back rubs and the Saturday night cheesecake run. But as labour starts, you will see just how pivotal your presence is in the childbirth process.

Being a Birth Partner

You'll wear a number of hats as birth partner – gofer, massage therapist, motivational speaker and lawyer. Your partner must focus completely on the task at hand, and she will rely on your support for quashing distractions and attending to her needs.

Don't be offended if you're told to take your stopwatch and shove it, or if she impatiently shoos you away as you try to regulate her breathing. She still wants you and, more importantly, needs you by her side. Be flexible, stick with it and work with her towards your common goal of a beautiful healthy baby.

Reassurance for the Faint of Heart

Birth, both by Caesarean and vaginally, can be a very blood-soaked scene. The chances are that the rush of seeing your baby emerge will overwhelm any aversions to blood and other bodily fluids. But if it doesn't, don't feel bad about taking a moment to collect yourself – outside the room if need be. A nurse or another support person can stand in for you in the meantime. Now is not the time to faint, fall and be concussed (although many an expectant dad has passed out in the heat of the moment). One tip – if you are known for getting the heebie-jeebies at the sight of blood, you and your partner should discuss the possibility of your early exit before labour. You may want to have a stand-by birth partner just in case.

If your partner is having a Caesarean, there will be a surgical curtain or drape positioned above her belly. Typically, dad is positioned by mum's head for emotional support throughout the procedure. To avoid the sight of blood and your partner's internal organs, simply stay below the sight line of the surgical drape by remaining seated on a stool by your partner's head. If the attending nurse hasn't given you a seat, ask for one.

The Best-Laid Plans

Things can go wrong in childbirth, but the more you know about any possible complications in advance, the easier it is to deal with them should they arise.

Emergency Birth

In cases where the foetus begins to show signs of distress (rapid acceleration or sudden slowdown of foetal heart rate) or you experience a life-threatening condition such as a haemorrhage, you will be rushed for an emergency Caesarean. In most cases, because time is of the essence, you will be given a general anaesthetic.

Women who attempt a vaginal birth after Caesarean (VBAC) may be at risk for uterine rupture or a separation of their previous Caesarean scar. If this occurs, an emergency Caesarean would be performed. It should be noted, however, that the success rate of VBAC is very good – between 60 and 80 per cent of individuals who are considered candidates for the procedure come through it with flying colours.

Delivery Complications

A child with a head too large for passage through the pelvis (called cephalopelvic disproportion), a labour that fails to progress past 6–7cm (2³/8–2³/4in) in spite of all efforts, or foetal distress caused by a compressed umbilical cord are all possible complications that could cause an unplanned Caesarean section.

In some cases, where your baby may need a little extra help getting out of the birth canal, the use of forceps may be required. This tong-like device is used to reach into the birth canal, gently grasp the baby's head, and pull him out. Forceps are also used to reposition a baby who is intent on arriving in a poor position.

Sometimes forceps are simply used to lift the baby up and out right there at your perineum, which is called perineal use or outlet forceps. Babies delivered via forceps wear signs of these instruments as bruises or red marks on either side of their heads for a few days, and there is a very slim risk of brain injury.

If your provider is concerned that using forceps will injure your perineal tissues, he may choose vacuum extraction instead. Suctioned onto the baby's head, a cup is attached to a chain that the doctor pulls on while you keep on pushing. The cup will simply fall off the baby's head if too much pressure builds up. However, babies who arrive via vacuum extraction can have a bruised, swollen look to the top of their heads – although this rights itself in time.

Other maternal complications may occur following a successful delivery. Postpartum haemorrhage and a related dive in blood pressure can occur when the uterus fails to contract again after both baby and placenta have been delivered. Compression and massage of the uterus and/or drug therapy may be used to stop the bleeding. In cases where a tear of the cervix has occurred, it will be sutured. If these measures still don't stop the bleeding, surgery may be required.

Chapter 19

Breast-feeding Basics

Breast-feeding is one part instinct, one part practice and a whole lot of persistence and patience. It's that last part that makes the difference between breast and bottle for many women, particularly in the first weeks of motherhood, when even minor nursing difficulties may seem insurmountable. The good news is that breast-feeding usually becomes easier and more fulfilling in time.

Breast or Bottle?

Are you going to breast-feed or go the formula route? It's an issue that many new mums feel intensely pressured about, and if you're still undecided, you've probably heard extensive opinions on the subject. Which is the right choice?

If you were comparing breast milk to formula strictly on a nutrient basis, few would disagree that the best choice is breast milk. But since the issue is also loaded with social, emotional and personal considerations, things are seldom so black and white. In the end, breast or bottle is an individual choice.

Pros and Cons

One woman's plus is another's 'no way'. Consider the pros and cons to breast- and bottle-feeding, and how they fit into your particular life and family situation.

Breast-feeding pros and cons

PRO: The hands-down perfect food for your child, breast milk is custom-made specifically for her nutritional needs and provides her with essential antibodies.
CON: If you have a medical condition that requires drug treatment, it's possible that your medication may pass into breast milk and potentially pose a risk to baby (talk to your doctor if this is the case; you may have other treatment options).

PRO: Breast-feeding is a low-maintenance feeding routine. It's always close at hand and never needs mixing, warming or other preparation.
CON: In the beginning, at least, you will always need to be close at hand as well. Breast-feeding can be as physically taxing as it is emotionally rewarding.

PRO: Nursing gives you special one-to-one bonding time with baby.
CON: Breasts don't detach. No one else can help with feeding duties.

PRO: If you're on a budget, breast-feeding is a big cost-cutter. Apart from the high cost of formula itself, you can save on bottles, bags, cleaning gadgets and other formula feeding purchases.
CON: You may have to purchase or hire a breast pump and buy a personal kit to use with it, which can also be costly.

PRO: As a breast-feeding mum, you're taking part in a tradition as old as motherhood itself and giving your child something no one else can. The experience is priceless.
CON: Unfortunately, there are still many unenlightened knuckleheads out there that can't get past their perception of the breast as strictly a sexual object and who will relegate you to the corner or better yet, the closet, if given the chance.

PRO: Many women who breast-feed experience faster postpartum weight loss.
CON: Although you may be getting your figure back, your breasts belong to baby, leaks, sore nipples and all.

Bottle-feeding pros and cons

PRO: Your partner can get up at 4 AM once in a while to feed the baby.
CON: The special mother-child bond and skin-to-skin contact that breast-feeding brings may be harder to achieve.

PRO: You can give your baby a bottle just about anywhere, at any time, without feeling self-conscious or raising eyebrows.
CON: Before you hit the road, make sure you've packed sterilized bottles and nipples, formula, bottled water for mixing powdered formula, a can opener for opening premixed formula, and an ice pack if you've made the bottles in advance. If they are chilled, you need a place to warm them, and don't forget the extra formula in case you're gone longer than you anticipated. Convenience is in the eye of the beholder.

PRO: No worries about keeping up your milk supply when you return to work.

CON: You may miss out on a golden opportunity to spend special nursing time together at home once your busy work schedule starts to encroach on family time again.

PRO: You can assume control of your body again, after many months away from the helm.

CON: After so many months as one, you're suddenly severing a close physical bond that nursing can prolong.

I can't nurse when I return to work in six weeks. Should I even bother breast-feeding, or will my baby get confused?
Even a short period of breast-feeding can have big advantages for your baby, so whatever time you can offer will be of benefit. However, completely and abruptly weaning him from the breast at six weeks will be hard for both of you. Bear in mind that many women return to work and continue to nurse, either by pumping or simply reducing the number of feedings from the breast so nursing is in the morning and the evening, and the baby is supplemented with formula at other times.

Being Comfortable with Your Decision

You are not an uncaring and self-absorbed mother if you choose to bottle-feed. Similarly, if you breast-feed your child openly and even through toddlerhood, you are not a mother-earth militant nutcase.

Try to weigh the risks versus the benefits in your situation. All other things being equal, women who are well-supported at home, are healthy and don't face an excessively demanding work schedule should consider giving breast-feeding a try, even if they feel a little awkward about it. Often the awkwardness evaporates with a little practice and the bond forged with baby in nursing. And the health benefits gained by baby will last a lifetime.

On the other hand, if you're a single mum who works two jobs and is already stretched to the limit emotionally and physically, don't be pressured into breast-feeding by others because it is 'the right thing to do'. Excessive stress can do more damage than good, impairing your parenting skills, putting your health at risk and straining the time the two of you do have together. Not every life situation is ideal for breast-feeding, even if you are capable of doing it. Make the decision that works best for your family.

Your Body and Breast-feeding

As soon as you can hold baby, you can breast-feed her. In the first few days following birth, your breasts will produce a clear to yellow sticky substance called colostrum, which contains antibodies that help strengthen the infant immune system. It also is important for getting baby's digestion on the right track. The low-carbohydrate, high-protein concoction is easily digestible for these early days and helps to establish intestinal flora, a beneficial bacteria, in baby's gastrointestinal tract. It also encourages the passing of meconium, your infant's first stools.

Colostrum comes out in small amounts compared to later breast milk, which will fill the alvoeli, or milk ducts, of your breast about three days after birth. You'll know when your milk 'comes in' – your breasts will become engorged with milk, rock-hard and sore to the touch. Nursing your baby will relieve the pressure quickly, although it's possible you may need a little additional help to ease soreness. A few clinical studies have shown some benefit in the use of cabbage leaves (yes, cabbage leaves) to relieve the discomfort of engorgement. Massage and warm compresses can also help.

tips

Sore or dry and cracked nipples are a common phenomenon as you get off the breast-feeding launch pad. Never fear – they will 'toughen up'. In the meantime, try vitamin E oil for moisturizing, or lanolin ointment for easing abrasions and pain. With the lanolin, a little goes a long, long way. You'll only need a tiny dollop on each nipple, and one tube will probably last you through infancy, toddlerhood and possibly beyond.

Latching and Letdown

Some babies seem to be breast-feeding champs from the start, and others need a little coaching. You're both new at this, so have patience and remember that you'll get better with practice. If you're having a hospital stay after your birth, the nurses on the maternity ward can give you some advice on technique and check baby's latching. In some cases, there may even be a lactation specialist on staff to consult.

Start with a comfortable position for the two of you. Baby's whole body should face yours, not just her turned head. The cradle and cross-cradle holds are two common positions. The cradle holds your baby close across the front of your body, with her head in the crook of your arm and your hand supporting her bottom. The cross-cradle switches arms and puts your hand under her head. Lying down with baby facing you is a good choice for the utterly exhausted.

The football position (or clutch hold) tucks baby under your arm, again facing your body and breast. If you've had a Caesarean, this can help by keeping the weight off your incision. It's also a favorite of mums with twins for doing double nursing duty (see Chapter 7 for tips on breast-feeding multiples). The seated Australian hold might be a good choice if you'd like to try to keep baby awake during and after his feeding. With all nursing positions, make sure your baby's head is well supported.

After you're settled into position, brace your breast with one hand, cupped into the shape of a 'C'. If you have small breasts, this may not be necessary after a time, but try the C-hold initially to make sure baby latches on correctly.

Encouraging baby to get a successful latch is the most important part of the process. Stroke her bottom lip with your nipple until she opens her mouth wide and yawn-like. This is called the rooting reflex. Insert your nipple into her mouth and she should instinctively close, or latch, onto it.

A proper latch:

- Encompasses the entire nipple and most, if not all, of the areola.
- Positions her nose almost directly on your breast (she can breathe, don't worry).
- Can be verified by her visible and possibly audible swallowing.
- Will *not* hurt (unless the nipple is in poor condition to begin with).

Cradle hold

◀ Choose a comfortable nursing position that works for both of you, and make sure baby's head is well-supported.

Cross-cradle hold

Football (or clutch) hold

Side lying hold

Australian hold

C-hold

◀ Use the C-hold to support your breast for baby and encourage a proper latch.

As your baby nurses, you'll feel a warm tingling that signals the milk ejection reflex (MER), or letdown. The feeling is actually milk being released into the sinuses of the breast for easy access by baby. Some women don't always feel the MER, but you'll know when it occurs if your baby suddenly picks up his pace of sucking and swallowing.

Supply-and-Demand System

When everything operates as designed, the more baby nurses, the more milk your breasts produce. A breast that baby has completely drained will produce milk at a faster rate than one that has only been partially emptiedy. Your milk production takes its cue from baby. So if your child is premature or ill and isn't nursing, or is latching or sucking ineffectively, your milk supply will adjust downwards. A breast pump can help keep the milk flowing until baby is ready to nurse full-time again.

Will this kid ever stop eating? It seems like I'm doing nothing but nursing!
Newborns don't believe much in schedules, do they? In some cases, constant nursing in a fussy baby might indicate an insufficient milk supply. But as long as he's growing well and is having six to eight wet nappies and about three dirty nappies daily, you can be assured he's getting plenty to eat. Nursing 10–12 times a day is also normal for a newborn. Just bear with it, and as the weeks pass and he develops, he'll spend more time exploring and less time eating. In the meantime, his frequent snacks are helping to establish and grow your milk supply, which is great.

Practical Matters

Button-up blouses, shirts with zips and other easy-access clothing will make nursing easier on a day-to-day basis. There are a variety of nursing bras available; make sure you try them on before purchase, to ensure a good fit. You may opt for the comfort of a jogging or sports bra that slides up easily, especially if you like the support of wearing a bra to bed.

Nursing pads for catching leaks before they soak through your shirt are also a must. These come in several different materials and configurations, including cloth, plastic and disposable – the latter have the advantage of high absorbency, while cloth can be washed and reused. Accidents do happen, even with pads, and carrying an extra shirt in your bag or car may save you a mortifying moment or two.

Every nursing mother could use a good breast-feeding reference book for guidance. Contact the La Leche League or the Natural Childbirth Trust (NCT) for further information.

Baby's Body and Breast-feeding

Trying to impose a strict feeding schedule on your newborn will result in much heartache and little success. Unless you have multiples, there's really no good reason to start scheduling baby's meals at specific times. If you do have twins or more, you may want to wake them all when one gets up for a feeding to get them on a similar routine, but that still doesn't mean feeding by the clock. Only your baby can determine how much he needs to satisfy his tummy, and feeding on demand is the best way to accomplish this.

The health rewards for your nursing child's body and mind are tremendous. Breast milk improves immunity, is thought to offer protection against certain chronic diseases (e.g. type 1 diabetes), is associated with a reduced risk of SIDS and is easy on baby's digestive system. Clinical studies have also indicated that breast-feeding may boost baby's brainpower and can enhance cognitive development in small for gestational age (SGA) babies.

So how long do you breast-feed for? The Department of Health recommends exclusive breast-feeding for six months, then breast-feeding until the baby is a year old. The best answer is probably as long as both of you are still enjoying and benefitting from it.

Bottle Basics

If you do choose to bottle-feed, there are literally hundreds of bottle types and teat configurations on the market. Figuring out what works and what doesn't is largely trial and error, but there are some things you can look for:

- **Low air flow.** Designs that minimize air or can be de-aired prior to feeding may reduce baby's wind.
- **Easy to clean.** Pick something with minimal parts that looks easy to clean and sterilize.
- **Built for baby.** Get a newborn-style teat with a smaller opening to start so baby doesn't face a formula tidal wave. If her sucking reflex is weak, you may have to upgrade to a larger opening.

f@ct

Baby's digestive system is still immature, and his tiny stomach can only hold 2–4 teaspoons of fluid at birth. For this reason, you'll notice spitting up is a frequent event. Don't be alarmed. It's his signal that the tank is full. Swallowing air and too much activity with a full tummy can also cause spitting up. However, if baby's spitting up becomes excessive and forceful (projectile vomiting), or is accompanied by gagging or difficulty swallowing, call your doctor immediately. It could be a sign that your baby has a formula intolerance or a gastrointestinal problem.

For women who are breast-feeding and need to introduce a bottle, look for a teat variety that mimics the natural contours of the breast. Your baby may be less likely to rejectt a bottle that feels similar to you.

Both breast-fed and bottle-fed babies require regular burping during a meal. You'll quickly pick up your child's cues that a bubble needs bursting; she may arch her back and fret at the breast or bottle. In the beginning, burping at least twice during a feeding session can help to ensure her comfort.

Seated

◀ There are several positions you can use to burp baby effectively: seated, over the shoulder and across the lap.

Seated

Over the
shoulder

Across the lap

Eating Well: For Mum

A pattern of healthy eating in pregnancy will continue to reward you and baby now that you're breast-feeding. Keep up the same routine with healthy food choices and plenty of non-caffeinated fluids (8–12 glasses a day).

Nursing burns approximately 500 calories per day, but that doesn't mean you will need to bulk out your diet significantly. Your body has plenty to spare and has stored extra fat for the very purpose of lactation. Note the modified breast-feeding mother's food pyramid.

▲ The modified food pyramid for breast-feeding mothers adds an extra serving from each food group.

Even though you may be tempted to cut calories drastically in order to get your old body back, now is not the time to crash-diet. Losing weight too quickly can release excessive levels of any toxins, such as pesticides and PCBs, that reside in your maternal fat stores, which will consequently pass into breast milk. Also stay away from extremely low-carbohydrate diets right now, as they can cause ketosis, another potential danger to a nursing baby.

On Your Mind

Breast-feeding doesn't come naturally to everyone. Ingrained feelings of self-consciousness about your body, of modesty and of discomfort with the process may inhibit your natural inclination to nurse. When things don't go according to plan and the nursing relationship isn't thriving, feelings of inadequacy are common. Seeking assistance, either through coaching or supplemental nutrition, is not a sign of failure, but rather of dedication to your child. Breast-feeding, in any amount, is something to take tremendous pride in.

Breasts: From Form to Function

Where is the right spot to nurse? Wherever your baby is hungry. As long as it's done as discreetly as circumstances warrant, there shouldn't be any place that's appropriate to bring a baby to that isn't also an appropriate place to breast-feed.

The thought of nursing in public may be worrying you. When the time comes, don't think about your exposure, think only of filling your child's stomach. A baby who's really singing for his supper will probably not give you the time to be modest about it, anyway.

Specially designed nursing blankets can improve your cover if you're really self-conscious, although a standard blanket over the shoulder works as well. If you do use one of these, make sure they're comfortable and not too hot for baby.

Support from Family and Friends

Breast-feeding doesn't always come naturally and immediately, particularly for first-time mums. Having the support of your friends and family is really important in making it through those first few uncertain and sometimes rocky weeks. Comments like 'Why don't you just give her a bottle?' will do nothing but erode your confidence and stress you . Get your partner's help in deflecting the negativity and explaining your reasons for breast-feeding, but if the bad attitudes continue, just avoid the offender. You don't need it.

A La Leche League group can also be a steadfast source of support and inspiration, and more importantly, guidance for your breast-feeding difficulties. Check the Yellow Pages for a local group.

Lactation Problems

Learning to read baby's body language and vocal cues is an acquired art, one that takes time to acclimatize to. It's easy to miss hunger signals, or mistake them for other needs. For now, familiarize yourself with the warning signs of insufficient feeding. If your baby is having fewer than six wet and three dirty nappies a day, is excessively fussy at the breast, has a sunken fontanelle (soft spot at the top of the head), is lethargic and is not at or above birth weight by two weeks postpartum (or steadily gaining thereafter), he is probably not getting enough, and needs to see the doctor immediately. Fortunately, with some work and a little guidance, you should both be able to get back on track.

Why Your Body Isn't Co-operating

There are dozens of reasons why milk supply or nursing itself may not be making the grade, but most of them can be overcome with patience, special equipment and/or professional training and guidance.

· **Medication:** Antihistamines, decongestants, contraceptives and some other medications can have a detrimental effect on milk supply. Talk to your doctor before taking any medication while nursing.

- **Inverted nipples:** If you have inverted nipples, a good latch may be elusive. Breast shields designed to pull the nipple out can help.
- **Prior breast surgery:** Many women nurse successfully after breast surgery, but certain types of breast-augmentation (enlargement) or breast-reduction surgery do have the potential to hinder your milk supply, depending on how they are performed. Talk to your doctor if you've had breast surgery and are having lactation problems.
- **Hypotrophic breast disease:** Some women have structural problems with the breast tissue that decreases the number of milk-producing ducts. You may still be able to nurse, but baby may require supplemental feedings. Again, speak to your doctor about your choices and options.
- **Retained placental fragment:** Lactation problems can be a sign that a piece of your placenta was missed in delivery. Since this can also cause severe haemorrhaginge, suspected retained placenta should be assessed by your doctor immediately.
- **Stress:** New motherhood and all its related stressors can inhibit milk supply, and tension can make letdown (milk ejection) difficult. If you're uptight about nursing problems, the cycle perpetuates itself. Try to look forward to nursing as a relaxing, *de*-stressing time.
- **Poor technique:** Letting baby empty one breast before moving on to the next will stimulate milk supply and allow her to reach the fatty and filling hindmilk that is at the end of her 'drink'.
- **Poor nutrition and hydration:** Good eating habits and plenty of water are essential to your milk-production efforts.
- **Nipple confusion:** The mechanics of drinking from a bottle are very different from those of feeding from the breast. If a bottle is introduced before breast-feeding is well established, it's possible for your baby to develop a preference for it.

Babies born prematurely, those with a poor sucking reflex or with a harelip or other health problems can have problems nursing initially. If your baby needs supplemental feeding in the hospital for any reason, you can ask for it to be administered with an eyedropper, syringe, feeding cup or supplemental feeding system, to avoid nipple confusion. You should also talk to your doctor and a lactation consultant about adaptive techniques and other options.

fact

Breast-feeding problems with your first baby may make you wary about trying it again. Keep in mind that just like every pregnancy and baby is different, nursing success can be too. Environmental factors play a large role in breast-feeding, so if the stress of your firstborn, coupled with the unprecedented exhaustion of that period, had your body in a tailspin, there's a good chance this time may be different. You also have the added benefit of experience on your side this time around. Don't be afraid to try again — if it doesn't work out, you still have options.

Lactation Consultants

A lactation consultant is a health care provider who specializes in breast-feeding support and training. If you're having difficulties with nursing, a consultant can be a huge help in helping you overcome breast-feeding difficulties. Your midwife or a health visitor can provide a referral if needed. Some pediatric practices retain lactation consultants on staff.

Many certified lactation consultants are also La Leche League leaders. Don't overlook the value of La Leche League support if you don't have a lactation consultant in your area. The organization can be a tremendous source of emotional support as well as practical advice and experience.

Pump Primer

A breast pump can be useful for increasing your milk production if you're having supply problems. It's also a great tool for mums heading back to work who want to keep nursing, and for mothers of babies who are temporarily unable to nurse because of various health issues.

A pump may be manual (hand-powered) or a battery or electric unit. The hand-powered pumps have the advantage of being inexpensive and portable, but may take some getting used to and take longer to empty a breast. They use a piston-like action or a squeeze bulb to create the suction that removes the milk from your breast.

Hospital-grade electric units are probably the most efficient and allow you to pump both breasts at the same time, but are bulky to transport and costly to purchase. Weekly or monthly hire units are frequently available through lactation consultants, hospital programmes or private businesses. For safety reasons, you will have to purchase a personal kit for use with the hired unit; this contains all the elements that come in contact with your breast milk, including tubing and bottles. The kit can be used for as long as you plan to pump.

Supplementing and Finger-Feeding

If you're having breast-feeding problems, a supplemental nursing system (SNS) can help you provide baby with added nutrients of pumped breast milk or formula while still getting the benefits of suckling. A bottle or bag milk reservoir hangs around your neck, and two narrow silicone tubes channel milk flow from the reservoir to your nipple, where the open end of the tube is taped. As baby feeds on both the supplemental milk and breast milk you're providing, her suckling action also further stimulates your milk production.

Women who are having problems producing enough milk, for whatever reason, may be able to supplement from a local breast milk bank. Milk donors are screened for health problems in a process similar to blood-donation screening. Again, a lactation consultant or paediatrician should have further information on what's available in your area.

Finger-feeding is similar in principle to an SNS, and is sometimes used as an alternative to an SNS. It uses a narrow feeding tube attached to a syringe or reservoir, in which breast milk or formula is placed. The other end of the tube is taped to your index or middle finger, and the baby gets her nourishment by sucking on your finger. If baby is not latching onto the breast for whatever reason (e.g. nipple confusion, separation from mum), finger-feeding can provide nutrition without introducing a rubber teat to the feeding process.

Mastitis

Mastitis is an infection of the breast that can be caused by a plugged milk duct. If you develop mastitis, you can, and should, keep nursing. Your baby cannot become ill from nursing from you during this time, and the breast-feeding process will actually help the mastitis resolve itself faster by easing the pain and draining the milk ducts.

Signs of mastitis include:
- Breast is warm to touch
- Red, tender streaks on the breast
- Pain and swelling
- Fever present

If you develop mastitis, stick to your nursing schedule and try to get sufficient rest to help your body heal. A warm water bottle, warm wet compress or soaking in a hot shower may help to ease the discomfort. If the mastitis doesn't start to clear up in a day or so, or begins to worsen, you may need an antibiotic. Your health-care provider can advise you as to what medications will be safe for breast-feeding. Putting fresh cabbage leaves in your bra can also relieve symptoms.

Just for Dads

Although it may look easy, breast-feeding can be hard work, particularly the first time. Your support is vital to this venture. Let your partner know you value this unique gift she's bestowing on your child. Be a voice of support when things get tough, and do what you can to create a warm and welcome environment for your nursing twosome. If you find the whole process bewildering, don't be embarrassed about asking questions.

Getting Comfortable with Breast-feeding

Be honest. Somewhere way in the back of your mind, or perhaps even at the front, you were a little freaked out at the concept of your partner as food source. If you weren't, more power to you, but it's normal to need a little time to adjust. Learning more about how beneficial breast-feeding is for your new baby may help increase your comfort level.

When you're both up to sex again, try to respect your partner's feelings about touching in the feeding zone. Nipple soreness, leaking milk and breast sensitivity may have her feeling best left alone. Or she may be willing and you may be hesitant, given whose mouth was there last. Whatever the situation, it's important you both get your current viewpoint out into the open so no one's feelings are hurt. Your outlook may evolve over time, or you may both decide to focus on other sources of pleasure.

One thing you'll quickly learn about infant timing is that you'll be interrupted in the heat of passion at least once. When she returns from nursing baby, realize that switching gears from nurturing mummy to adventurous sex kitten can be a tall order to fill. Don't force the uncomfortable and awkward if the moment has passed for either of you. You won't have an infant forever, and this is just one of the many sudden detours of life that being a parent brings.

Getting in on the Act

Just because your partner may be nursing doesn't cut you out of the feeding picture completely. At some point, after breast-feeding has been established, you will want to familiarize baby with a bottle of breast milk, in case mum's absence requires feeding her expressed milk.

Once a bottle is introduced, you can do the honours for a regular feeding. Some babies are hesitant to take a bottle from mum when they know her nice warm breast is just an arm's reach away, so your presence may be a necessity for this task.

Chapter 20

Bringing Baby Home

The first days at home with your new family are fun but challenging. Your body is going through some intense physical changes. And if you thought those hormonal changes that pregnancy brought were now finished, well, think again. Enjoy this special time of getting acquainted and settling into your new lifestyle.

Your Body Postpartum

From the moment your child slides out of your body, a transformation as dramatic as that of pregnancy begins. At delivery you will drop around 4.5–6.7kg (10–15lb) of baby, placenta, amniotic fluid and lochia.

By the tenth day postpartum, your incredible shrinking uterus will have contracted to one-twentieth of its size before labour, and the cervix will be closed once again. Afterpains similar to menstrual cramp and a steady discharge of lochia indicate that the uterus is returning to normal. The lochia flow will continue for up to six weeks, but the afterpains will probably stop several days after delivery (although nursing may continue to stimulate them periodically).

Your perineal area may continue to be sore for a few weeks, particularly when you need to relieve yourself. Take your peribottle from the hospital home with you and keep it in the toilet for regular use. A hot water bottle and occasional cold packs can also ease pain and swelling. If sitting is uncomfortable, you can purchase a foam cushion for your chair at a medical supply store. Most stitches dissolve within a week, and external ones may fall out. Pelvic floor exercises can help speed up the healing process.

tips

Lochia flow will be heavy and bright red at first, but the colour will gradually change to pink and then yellow or brown. The flow will taper off within 10–14 days, although some discharge is normal for up to six weeks. However, the bright red colour may begin again at times. If it does, take it as a sign that you may be doing too much too soon, and slow down. Never use tampons to control lochia flow because of the risk of infection.

As your body drops tissue and fluids, and decreases its cardiovascular volume, your metabolism may seem completely out of kilter. Vaginally, things may seem a little 'looser' in general. Your vaginal skin is quite elastic, and may be stretched from the birth. Exercise and time will help it return to a firmer state.

Constipation is another common postpartum problem, primarily because of the loss of abdominal muscle tone and painkillers that can slow your digestive processes. Plenty of water, movement and high-fibre foods may help. If you had a Caesarean, your incision may also make you hesitant to bear down very hard. Supporting it with a rolled-up towel can help. A stool softener may be prescribed as well; check with your doctor before taking any medication if you are breast-feeding.

Your breasts will be tender as you deal with engorgement. Women who aren't planning to nurse will find that drying up your milk supply fully can be a somewhat uncomfortable process. If you do breast-feed, sore nipples and other discomforts may plague you as you adjust to this new routine.

Recovering after a Caesarean

When you've had a Caesarean you're recovering from major surgery and need to treat yourself accordingly. Sleep when baby sleeps, and stay away from strenuous activity and heavy lifting (nothing bigger than baby as a general rule, and certainly not a full baby bath). Use a bed pillow or a nursing pillow to hold your baby without pressuring your incision. Pain medication may be prescribed; if you're breast-feeding, talk to your doctor about judicious use.

Your doctor will recommend six weeks of rest and recuperation (within limits – you are a new mum, after all), and you'll be advised not to drive while taking pain medications. Second or subsequent Caesarean mums may recover a bit quicker, just because they know what to expect and treat themselves accordingly. Above all, don't push it, or you'll set your recovery back even further.

Women can and do get pregnant in the period following birth. Although sex may be the last thing on your mind at the moment, if you aren't up to a return to the delivery room in nine or ten short months, get back on a contraceptive routine now before the mood strikes. Your doctor can give you a prescription before you leave the hospital, if necessary.

Baby's Body: An Operator's Manual

Your baby will actually lose weight as she starts out in life, but should be back up to birth weight by her two-week checkup. Thereafter, she may put on 454g (1lb) every two weeks, doubling her birth weight by month 4. Premature babies sometimes grow a little slower, but most will eventually catch up.

Her eyesight is a bit hazy, but she can see you fairly clearly when you hold her 178–255mm (7–10in) away from your face. Studies show she knows your voice well already from listening to it in the womb, and prefers it to a stranger's.

Your newborn arrives with a variety of natural reflexes or involuntary ways of moving:

- **Palmar, or grasping, reflex.** When you touch your baby's open hand, she'll make a fist around your finger.
- **Rooting reflex.** If you stroke her cheek, her head will turn toward your touch. This reflex helps the bleary-eyed newborn find her food source, and you can use it to guide her to the breast or bottle.
- **Sucking reflex.** Once at the breast or bottle, baby's sucking reflex takes over as she automatically sucks on anything put in her mouth.
- **Startled, or moro, reflex.** When baby is startled, he will thrust his arms and legs out and arch his back, then quickly pull arms and legs in again.
- **Babinski reflex.** Stroking baby's foot will make him spread his toes and flex his foot in.
- **Stepping reflex.** Hold your baby up with your hands under her armpits so that her feet are touching a firm surface. She will lift her feet up and down like she is about to take baby steps.
- **Tonic neck reflex.** When placed on his back, baby turns his head to the right and makes fists with his hands.
- **Blinking.** The involuntary reflex of closing her eyes when they are exposed to bright light, air or another stimulus is the one reflex that baby will keep for the rest of her life.

From Soft Spot to Curled Toes

The bones of baby's skull are not yet fused together, and unless you had a Caesarean delivery, your baby's head may look a bit, well, pointed. This cone-headed appearance is the result of pressure in the birth canal and will round out within a few weeks. There are four small areas on your baby's head where the baby's skull bones have not yet joined together, called fontanelles (or soft spots). Three of these fontanelles fuse within the first four months of life, but the longest lasting and most visible of these – the diamond-shaped area on the top of the head, called the anterior fontanelle (or soft spot) – may take up to 18 months to close. Many a curious sibling has reached out to jab this pulsating spot, much to their parent's horror. Don't get too concerned – your baby's brain is well protected by a tough membrane called the dura mater.

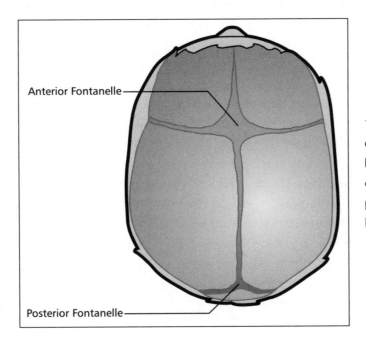

Anterior Fontanelle

Posterior Fontanelle

◄ Baby's soft spot is called a fontanelle. She has a total of four, but only the anterior and posterior are easily located.

The eye colour your baby has at birth may change later in infancy or childhood. This is due to the ongoing production of the hormone melanin, which can cause later eye-colour changes.

If the fontanelle ever appears deeply sunken or bulging, call the doctor immediately. A sunken soft spot is a sign of dehydration, or your baby not getting sufficient fluids. And a fontanelle that bulges could be an indication of increased pressure in the brain from fluid build-up or haemorrhage. Keep in mind that crying can make the fontanelle appear swollen. A normal fontanelle is slightly curved in and soft yet firm to the touch.

Baby's Skin

Your newborn's soft-as-butter skin may have some imperfections at first. Post-term babies are more likely to have some peeling, while preterm babies may still be sporting a substantial amount of lanugo and vernix. Although the vernix is fairly well rubbed off by the time you bring baby home, you may continue to find it in his creases and crevices until his first real bath. The lanugo will rub itself off over the next few weeks.

Baby may also be wearing one or more birthmarks on his birthday suit. Red marks on the eyelids, forehead and very back of the nape of the neck usually fade and disappear over time and are called salmon patches or stork bites. Red, strawberry birthmarks can increase in size, but may shrink and be gone by age five. Your baby may also have one or more light brown birthmarks known as café au lait spots. Very rarely, café au lait spots (particularly many marks) are symptomatic of one of several uncommon medical conditions. Talk to your doctor about any concerns.

Dark blue to blue-green spots on the buttocks or lower back are known as Mongolian spots. They are most common in Afro-Caribbean and Asian newborns, and fade over time. If your baby is born with what is known as a port wine stain, a bright red or purple mark that is considered to be more permanent, plastic surgery is an option in later life if they are located in a prominent spot. Ask your paediatrician or family doctor for more information.

Little whiteheads called milia are common on newborns, and you may see them around the nose. Caused by oil-secreting glands, the pimples may come and go during the first few days. You may also see petechia, red to purple pinpoints, on baby's face from the trauma of coming down the birth canal. These will disappear in a few days as well.

Your boy or girl may have swollen breasts that actually leak milk. This milk, known in folk medicine as 'witch's milk', is the product of your pregnancy hormones at work on your newborn. Avoid massaging the area, as this can trigger an abscess. The breats will return to normal size within a few days.

The Umbilical Cord

Baby's umbilical cord stump looks just like it sounds, a dark, dried-up protrusion. Since it is basically dead tissue, it is black in colour. You'll be instructed to clean it regularly, usually with swabs, and keep it dry to prevent breakage and bleeding. Keep an eye open for signs of infection, such as pus or inflammation. Within two weeks or so, the stump will fall off and your baby's perfect little belly button will be revealed.

Genitals

Before your partner congratulates himself too heartily on your well-endowed son, you may want to break the news that it is probably just a passing phenomenon. Newborn boys and girls are often born with swollen genitals, again due to the effects of your pregnancy hormones working on them. Girls may even have a bit of mucus discharge, possibly blood-tinged, from their vaginas.

Fingernails and Toenails

Baby's tiny curled fingers and toes usually emerge in need of a manicure. Growing for several months in the womb, they are typically long and ragged. The thought of trimming such tiny appendages may fill you with dread, but it's not as hard as you might think. Just make sure you have the right tools (infant-sized clippers), and try to trim while baby is sleeping if you'd like to avoid wrestling with a moving target. If you still can't seem to get it right, bring your clippers with you to your two-week appointment and ask for advice.

Sleeping Like a Baby

In the beginning, it will seem like your little one is sleeping quite a bit. In fact, she's snoozing for up to 18 hours a day. If she's your first, you may be crouched outside her door waiting to run in and get some quality play time at the first rustle (second-time parents, on the other hand, count down the minutes to nap time). While her sleep patterns, which involve four-hour stretches of snoozing, won't have a huge effect on your day schedule, they're going to hit you hard at night. She'll be waking up to be fed several times an evening for at least the first three months.

Remember to always place your baby on his back when laying him down for a nap or bedtime. Back sleeping has been shown to reduce the incidence of sudden infant death syndrome, or SIDS. Make sure baby's crib is clear of stuffed animals, quilts, pillows and other soft bedding when he heads to bed as well.

◀ Baby should always be put to sleep on his back. If a thin blanket is necessary, place baby with his feet at the bottom end of the crib and make sure the blanket is tucked in between mattress and crib and goes no higher than baby's chest.

Postpartum Depression

Feeling down is a common postpartum emotion that typically passes in a few weeks. For many women, however, these feelings go beyond the basic baby blues and signal a more serious depressive or endocrine disorder.

The Baby Blues

The majority of new mothers experience what has commonly become known as the 'baby blues', a short-lived period of mild depression that appears in up to 85 per cent of postpartum women. A severe shortage of sleep, disappointment with the birth experience, see-sawing hormone levels, anxieties about baby's health and well-being, and shaky confidence in your own parenting skills can all lead to feelings of sadness and inadequacy. Fortunately, most cases of the blues resolve themselves within a few days to two weeks after birth, as balance returns to the new mother's life.

When It's More Than the Blues

More serious is postpartum depression (PPD), which occurs in about 10 per cent of new mothers, and can drag on for up to a year. If you're experiencing one or more of the following symptoms, talk to your doctor about PPD:

- Feelings of extreme sadness and inexplicable crying jags
- Lack of pleasure in things you would normally enjoy
- Trouble concentrating
- Excessive worrying about the baby or, conversely, a lack of interest in the baby
- Feelings of low self-esteem
- Decreased appetite

Fortunately, PPD can be effectively treated with counselling and/or antidepressant drugs, so ask your doctor for a referral to a mental health professional. Even if you're breast-feeding, you may have medication options; there are several antidepressant drugs on the market that are thought to have minimal effects on nursing infants. A number of studies involving sertraline (Zoloft), for example, found that while the drug passes into breast milk, the levels it reaches in the nursing infant were clinically insignificant, in some cases too low to even be detected in standard laboratory blood tests.

Safety cannot be guaranteed, however; studies on how antidepressants might affect a breast-fed child in the long term are not available. On the other hand, clinical research has demonstrated a measurable detrimental effect on children of depressed mothers when PPD goes untreated. Each woman must evaluate the risks of treatment versus the benefits when deciding if drug therapy is right for them.

Postpartum Psychosis

One in every 1,000 women experiences a severe form of PPD known as postpartum psychosis (or puerperal psychosis). Symptoms include hallucinations, delusions, contemplation of hurting oneself or others, insomnia and turbulent mood swings. Postpartum psychosis is a medical emergency that needs immediate treatment and usually hospitalization. The good news is that with proper care, full recovery can be expected.

Thyroid Problems

Thyroid problems are fairly common after childbirth, but the symptoms can be confused with other postpartum conditions. Milk supply difficulties, extreme fatigue, hair loss, depression, mood changes, problems losing weight or unusually rapid weight loss, heart palpitations, menstrual irregularities and sleep disorders are all common signs of postpartum thyroid conditions.

If you're experiencing signs of postpartum depression, make sure your doctor tests your thyroid levels. Up to 10 per cent of new mothers experience thyroid problems following childbirth, and the typical symptoms of fatigue, depression and unexplained weight loss can mimic postpartum depression.

Some women have temporary postpartum hyperthyroidism – an overactive thyroid, with weight loss, diarrhoea, racing heart, anxiety and other symptoms of a revved up metabolism. Doctors may prescribe drugs to ease symptoms, but this condition often resolves itself quickly.

Other women can develop temporary postpartum hypothyroidism – an underactive thyroid – with fatigue, weight gain, constipation, depression and other symptoms of a slowed-down metabolism. Again, medication may be prescribed, depending on the severity of symptoms, and frequently the thyroid will return to normal within six months to a year after the birth.

New mothers with a family or personal history of autoimmune or thyroid disease may benefit from routine thyroid testing in the first month postpartum. It can be hard to tell what's 'normal' after having a baby, but if any of the above symptoms become debilitating, a thyroid test can quickly rule out or diagnose a thyroid problem.

Women who experience temporary postpartum thyroid problems are at a higher risk to develop thyroid disease later in life, and should talk to their doctor about regular follow-up screening.

Adjusting to Your New Schedule

Many aspects of your life will be different now that you are a parent. You may feel that your priorities are very different now that you have a little one. But taking time to care for yourself is equally important.

Bonding with Baby

These early weeks and months are a precious time of getting to know each other and building confidence. Yet, as she's cried for 20 minutes straight and you still haven't guessed what's wrong (is she hungry, dirty, tired, colicky, windy?), you may start to wonder about your mothering abilities. Trust yourself. It takes time to learn her language, but the patience and persistence you invest in decoding her signals will pay off. You'll crack the code eventually, and in the process you'll establish a bond of trust and communication that will last a lifetime.

The term 'bonding' was coined in 1976 by Drs Marshall Klaus and John Kennell, two professors of paediatrics who published *Maternal-Infant Bonding*. Klaus and Kennell introduced the theory that close, personal contact between mother and baby was essential in the first 30–60 minutes after birth to build the foundation for a healthy attachment.

Sleep, or Lack of It

People told you how tired you would be when baby arrived, but after three months of uncomfortable and interrupted sleep leading up to the delivery, you thought you were well prepared. Surprise. You feel like the walking dead, and crave sleep constantly. Your baby will sleep through the night eventually. In the meantime, give yourself a break by splitting night duties with your partner. Even if you're breast-feeding, if baby is in another room he can help out by retrieving and returning her. Also remember the new mum motto: 'Nap when the baby naps.' Forget laundry, forget dishes. You need your rest more than a clean house right now.

And if you've only slept three hours last night between bouts of calming a fussy baby? Don't get behind the wheel of a car before you get some adequate shuteye. Extreme fatigue slows your reaction time and you run a very real risk of falling asleep behind the wheel. The National Highway Traffic Safety Administration (NHTSA) estimates that driving while drowsy is responsible for at least 100,000 automobile accidents annually between the hours of 10 PM and 6 AM.

Setting Priorities

You aren't going to be able to do it all. If you try to keep up your pre-parenthood schedule in addition to your new motherhood duties, something or someone has got to give. Usually it's your sanity. Things that just aren't that important, and usually anything in the domesticity arena can lag behind a bit. As the motivational gurus like to say, work smarter, not harder. Buy the birthday cake at the bakery instead of baking it yourself. Use a delivery service to get your shopping. Pay the kid from down the street to mow the lawn.

Don't Forget to Have Fun

Once you get past the fatigue, the uncertainties and the occasional frustrations, being a new mum can be incredibly entertaining. You have a legitimate excuse to play, explore, rhyme, sing and revisit your childhood in general. You have an adoring little person who hangs on your every word and movement and loves you unconditionally. And you get to witness all her incredible firsts as your tiny miracle learns to smile, roll over, crawl and eventually walk and talk. In a year, this postpartum time will be a distant memory. Treasure it while it's here.

The Rest of the Family

Obviously, you aren't doing this alone. Even if you're a single mum, you have people in your life who care for you and baby. Involve your family or those around you, and baby and you will benefit.

Support

You might learn that your mother really does know a thing or two. It's amazing to watch her and your dad soothe and burp their grandchild as if they had only been doing it yesterday - just like riding a bike, apparently, and they often have a baby-soothing trick or two up their sleeve that will make your life easier. Every family relationship is different, of course, but witnessing someone who raised you cuddle and care for the child that you will now nurture instills a sense of connectivity and completeness, as if your life has come full circle. Now just hope that all those prophecies they made about 'hoping you have a child just like you' don't come to fruition!

Neighbours and friends will probably call, both to check on the new addition and find out if they can do anything for you. One simple rule: take all help that is offered. Don't feel guilty, don't feel as though you're putting anyone out. They wouldn't offer if they didn't mean it. And if they offered just because they thought they should, they'll think twice next time, won't they?

What's the best way to introduce a dog and new baby to each other?

Pets can be a wonderful influence in your child's life and create many happy memories, but only if they're properly supervised and trained. Because animals learn so much from scents, some new parents bring home a blanket that smells like the new baby and give it to their dog to get acquainted. Let their first meeting be a gradual and calm affair, with only immediate family present. And remember, even if you have the most mild-mannered pet in the world, you need to preside over all his encounters with your child. It only takes a split second for baby to grasp a handful of fur and cause your pet to go on the defensive.

Sibling Rivalry

Give your older child a chance to bond with baby on the sibling level as well. Older kids frequently get a kick out of holding, feeding and 'protecting} their new little sister or brother. Children of nursery-school age or younger may have a more difficult time accepting this drain on their parents' attention. Some tips to promote sibling harmony:

- If you're breast-feeding, establish a family routine of a snack or story when baby nurses, to make it a special time for all.
- Involve your child in age-appropriate baby care. Helping with a bath or nappy change may be just the incentive they need to relish their new big brother or sister role.
- Try to arrange some special parental one-to-one time. Even if it's just a quick story during baby's nap, try to have a designated time where your firstborn is the star of the show.
- Tell your older child stories about their babyhood. Hearing how they threw strained peas at daddy or wore their very ripe nappy as a hat will have them in stitches and may help them relate to this odd little creature a bit better.
- Don't use the baby as an excuse. If they hear 'We can't do that because

the baby is sleeping' constantly, guess who they will start to blame for the new hurdle in their social life? Instead, provide baby-friendly alternatives when you say no: 'We can't go swimming today, but we can go for a walk to the park.' And arrange some time to take your 'big kid' someplace he's been dying to go without a sibling in tow.

Daddy Time

Don't hog the baby. Make sure that daddy gets his own chance at bonding time. With a constant flow of visitors and your many hours clocked on baby duty, he may be feeling left out. Both he and your child need time alone together. Getting out and moving for a short walk is good exercise for you now and a good way to clear your head after a day of talking in babyspeak. Hand the reins over, without direction or judgment if at all possible, and give dad a chance to run the show.

Just for Dads

Finally, a chance for hands-on parenting. Yet you may still find yourself feeling outside the family circle. Are you hesitant to jump into this foreign world, or are you feeling like there isn't much left for you to handle? Remember that it is just as important for you to forge a strong bond with your child as it is for your partner. Start small if it helps your confidence level. Even a task as simple as changing your baby is an opportunity for relationship building.

Developing Your Own Daddy Style

There is more than one right way to change a nappy, warm a bottle and calm a fretful baby. You will have your own way of doing things, and that is more than all right, that's good for your whole family. It teaches your baby that there are differences between mummy and daddy, and she will learn what to expect from your unique parenting style.

Don't be a bystander. If you feel like you're getting the brush-off when it comes to baby, let your partner know. She may be so preoccupied with new motherhood and other concerns that she isn't even aware she's doing it.

Offer to take charge of regular tasks like bathing. If you feel a little unsure, ask mum to stay within shouting distance so you can get help if need be. But remember, the only reason she seems to handle baby so effortlessly is practice. That's all you need as well.

Set up a date for just baby and you – a trip to the park, a neighbourhood walk, even some playtime in the back garden will do. Your partner can have some badly needed time to herself, and you can stretch your care-giving wings.

Male Bonding

You are smitten, preoccupied, utterly in love with this new person in your life, and she with you. The feeling is aptly called engrossment, and it's your version of dad-to-baby bonding. Despite society's expectations and dated clichés of fatherhood, men can be just as nurturing and loving parents and caregivers as women. So dote on your child, spend time with her, play with her, change her, tickle her and do whatever comes naturally.

Easing Back into Intimacy

Once baby arrived and your wife got at least a shadow of her former self back, you thought sex would quickly follow. It hasn't. When you lay out the realities, it shouldn't surprise you. Quick snatches of sleep, a sore and still recovering body, and all the concerns and anxieties that come with new motherhood are putting the damper on intimacy yet again.

If she is the primary caregiver at home with baby right now, there may be days when she doesn't even manage to get her clothes on until well past noon. Having dried spit in your hair and baby poo on your pyjama bottoms doesn't make you feel much like getting romantic. She needs a little empathy, TLC and pampering (yes, again) to get back into a more amorous state of mind. Work on supporting her, helping with household duties, and encouraging her rest and recovery. Once her basic physical needs are met, she can spend a little more time on the two of you.

Chapter 21

Back in the Swing of Things

Although it seems overwhelming at first, it won't take you long to get the parenting basics down. Making career and family choices, building new and stronger relationships with your partner, and getting back in tune with your body are all priorities during the first year postpartum.

Getting Your Body Back

Another time-worn motherhood maxim that is worth repeating: it took nine months for you to look this way, so give yourself at least that much time to get your body back. Actually, giving yourself a year is perhaps more realistic if you work in a three-month transitional period after the birth of your child. As you hammer out a routine where you and baby can manage to get dressed and bathed before dinnertime, you won't have much time for structured exercise in those early days.

Set realistic goals for weight loss. Losing weight too rapidly can actually be dangerous for you, and for your child if you're breast-feeding, since you need 500 extra calories per day for nursing. In general, most women need to lose about another 4.5kg (10lb) to return to their pre-pregnant weight at their six-week postpartum visit. Many women find it difficult to lose weight during this period because they're working hard, nursing and sleep-deprived. The time crunch all new mothers face can make a sensible and nutritious diet and regular exercise seem like a monumental task. Start slowly and easily, and the rest will follow.

Stretch marks—your merit badges of pregnancy—are not going to disappear with exercise. If they haven't already, they will probably fade to barely noticeable silvery squiggles, and no one but you will probably even recognize them. But if you are self-conscious, studies have show that both Retin-A and laser treatment are effective methods for banishing them. Ask your doctor for further information, and if you're breast-feeding, make sure you let your doctor know so he can prescribe treatment and medications accordingly.

Exercise

Once you have your doctor's OK to get moving again, start slowly. Even if you were a fitness fanatic throughout pregnancy, you'll still have to work to reach your former level of condition. Listen to your body. If you experience bright red lochia discharge, it's a signal that you're probably doing too much, too fast.

If you've had a Caesarean, it's really important to stick to the doctor's orders regarding exercise. Most providers will recommend at least a six-week recovery time, but talk to your doctor about guidelines specific to you. Don't risk your health by starting a fully fledged campaign for your pre-pregnancy body before that time.

Many new mums find that their biggest challenge to regular exercise is just finding the time. Try these tips for squeezing it in:

- **Keep it simple.** Programmes with steps, balls, bands, saucers and other gear are probably not for you right now if you're just getting started. You haul around enough stuff just keeping baby clean and well-fed. Don't add to it.
- **Baby steps.** Start small. Commit yourself to 20–30 minutes a day of movement, and work your way up from there.
- **Pencil yourself in.** Set a regular schedule for your partner or a babysitter to care for baby, and use the time to get out and get yourself up and moving.

f@ct

Many childhood education programmes and community centres offer parent and child exercise classes, so check out this fun way to teach your child healthy fitness habits early on. If there are no classes in your neck of the woods, try one of the many kids' or child-parent exercise videos or DVDs on the market. Check your local library or film-hire shop first so you can find one you like before buying.

- **Be flexible.** Do away with the all-or-nothing attitude. If you can't get to the gym one day, take a brisk walk or bike ride instead. Every little bit helps.
- **Friend system.** If you're lucky enough to have a friend or neighbour nearby who is also a new mum, pair up. You can cheer each other on and commiserate.
- **Get baby in on the act.** Get a jogging buggy and start a regular walking schedule, or simply incorporate more activity into your play. The park is a great place to start.

• **Join a gym.** Many health clubs and community programmes have nursery areas for their members. This may be an option for you if it is financially feasible. Do take the opportunity to watch the staff in action before enrolling.

Eating Properly

Exercise and good nutrition together are the best way to lose your pregnancy weight. If you established healthy eating patterns in pregnancy, you're ahead of the game. If not, now is as good a time as any to get started.

Breast-feeding shouldn't change your diet substantially. Some doctors may advise a slight caloric increase of around 500 calories daily to meet milk production needs, but others believe no increase is necessary. Talk to your doctor for specific guidance.

Another big benefit of breast-feeding can be a faster postpartum rate of weight loss. Although every mum is different, nursing helps you drop fat stores you collected in pregnancy for the very purpose of lactation. Your body works hard to produce milk, and also burns calories faster as a result.

If you had gestational diabetes during your pregnancy, you have a higher risk of developing insulin resistance and type 2 diabetes. The British Diabetes Association recommends that your blood glucose levels be tested six weeks after pregnancy, and at subsequent three-year intervals thereafter (more frequently if you show signs of impaired glucose tolerance postpartum). Fortunately, lifestyle modifications such as exercise and weight loss are very effective at preventing these conditions.

Typically, as long as you're choosing your foods wisely, you can let your stomach be your guide. Drink plenty of fluids. They're essential to keeping you well hydrated, and nursing has a tendency to make you thirsty. Having a glass of water or other non-caffeinated beverage each time baby nurses is a good ritual to establish proper fluid intake. The restrictions of pregnancy (no alcohol, tobacco, etc.) should also be continued throughout breast-feeding.

Making Up Sleep Deficits

Sleep is also an important factor in getting your old self back. If you're too tired to function, exercise has little appeal. You may find yourself opting for a fast-food fix for dinner instead of taking the time and energy to prepare healthier fare. And your health can suffer as well. Sleep deprivation affects the immune system; chronic sleep loss has been linked to decreases in growth hormone (responsible for bone marrow growth and tissue healing); increased insulin resistance; and a decline in tumour necrosis factor (or natural killer cells; cancer and virus fighting agents). Mood disorders, such as depression, can also be made worse by insufficient sleep. And, of course, you're already aware of the zombie-like brain fog that those all-nighters bring. In short, sleep loss is a real health hazard. You can't run on empty forever.

So how do you get it back? Take naps whenever possible, of course, and consider a little creative shift work. If your child is not nursing when he wakes in the middle of the night, you can switch off night-shift baby duty with dad so at least one of you has unbroken slumber every other day. This is even possible with breast-feeding if you've introduced a bottle to baby. Just pump breast milk the evening before so your presence won't be necessary. You may get a protest the first time dad attempts to put baby back to sleep with a rubber teat instead of mum's warm breast, but don't give up on the first try. Sometimes a little adjustment period is all that's necessary to ease into this new schedule.

The Incredible Changing Baby

Your infant will reach new milestones in such dizzying succession that you'll be convinced you have a prodigy on your hands. Watch her transform from a floppy-necked, bleary-eyed newborn to an active and alert infant in a matter of months. As she starts to become more aware of her surroundings and interact more with you and her environment, providing encouragement, stimulation and patience will help her thrive.

Your doctor will give you an idea of appropriate developmental milestones as your baby grows. Remember, these are just averages, and some may be reached earlier and/or later than others. Every child grows at his own pace. The main function of milestones is to serve as a screening tool; if baby is lagging on many it may be a sign of a problem, but one or more delays are typically no cause for concern.

Premature growth and development are assessed based on the age from estimated delivery date instead of actual birth date for the first two years of life. So a four-month-old infant who was born one month prematurely would be assessed for her attainment of three-month developmental milestones and size guidelines instead of four-month milestones.

Your Career

As maternity leave approaches its end, you may find yourself faced with decisions you hadn't anticipated. The thought of leaving baby with a childminder could be tearing you apart. Conversely, if you've put your career on hold for now to stay home with your child, you may find yourself missing the mental challenges and feelings of self-validation provided by work. Changing your mind, either for or against a career outside the home, is not a terrible thing.

If You Decide Not to Return to Work

You had every intention of going back to the office after maternity leave was over, but you never expected to fall so deeply in love with not just your child, but motherhood. Or perhaps it's the thought of leaving your vulnerable little infant with someone outside his immediate family that has you rethinking your options.

Financial concerns are an issue, of course. In many cases, the costs of child care and career-related expenses, such as dry-cleaning bills and transport costs, can come close to offsetting the difference between a one- and two-income lifestyle.

There may be a middle ground – picking up part-time work to cover the spread – or getting dad to stay at home may be a viable alternative. Sit down and thrash out the numbers with your partner. Flexibility and creative thinking may reveal a solution.

Going Back to Work

One of the hardest parts of new parenthood is heading back to the office. Getting up to speed on projects and procedures, handling the deluge from managers and colleagues who were basically lost without you, and fighting to stay off the 'mummy track' – all while worrying about how your child is adapting to her new care arrangements – is a tall order to handle. If you can arrange it, try easing back into things with a reduced schedule (half days or three days a week) to smooth the transition for both of you. Chapter 9 has more information and advice on returning to work as a new mum, as well as breast-feeding basics for the office.

How can I find good child care?
Your best source of leads for good child care is other mums in your life who share your values and viewpoints on child-rearing. You can narrow down your list to facilities that have adequate staffing (for infants, this is generally a minimum of one provider to every three babies), a stimulating and child-friendly environment, and caring and nurturing staff. Proper licensing and accreditation are also important.

Making Time for Yourself, and Using It

When your career gets back in the picture, things can accelerate to a frenzied pace. Don't just pay lip service to the idea of making time for yourself; do it. Even though it may be incredibly tempting to cancel your grown-up plans in favour of lazing around at home or getting some extra household chores done, don't give in to the temptation. You'll find time alone or with adult company (work doesn't count) is a great recharger. Here are some tips for following through.

- **Buy tickets to something.** You're less likely to bow out if there's money involved.

- **Invite a friend.** Again, committing to a date and event will make you more likely to follow through.
- **Pick something with a payoff.** A shopping trip to the one place where you know they have that hard-to-find Christmas gift you've been searching for may get you up and out.
- **Schedule a babysitter right from the start.** A short respite from child care, particularly if it leaves baby in the hands of a doting relative who would be sorely disappointed if you cancelled, is a good incentive to keep your date with yourself.

A Whole New Family

In addition to your new relationship, other family dynamics have definitely changed since baby's arrival. You and your partner may find yourselves hard-pressed for time to spend together, and practical matters like money may be more of an issue as you learn how to adjust your lifestyle and income for three (or more). If you have some specific goals for family planning, you may even be thinking about pregnancy again.

Intimacy Issues

Perhaps for the first time in months, you may be rediscovering your interest in sex. Of course, your little one may be putting a damper on things unwittingly – rest assured, she is bound to interrupt you in the height of passion at least once. Flexibility is the key to having a healthy sex life with kids around. Grab time together when it presents itself, and follow these tips for rekindling the fire:

- **No baby talk.** Calling each other 'Mummy' and 'Ddaddy' around the kids is fine, but it can really kill the mood if it slips out in other circumstances.
- **Take it slow and easy.** Give both of you time to rediscover each other. There may be a learning curve with your post-pregnancy body.
- **Love yourself.** It's hard to enjoy lovemaking if you're self-conscious about the way you look. Accept the state of your body, whatever it is,

and see it instead as a visible symbol of the miracle of your baby.

- **Quiet, please.** You don't need to turn the baby monitor up to 11. Hearing every tiny baby sigh is a turnoff. Just turn the monitor down or open your door instead; if she wakes up, she will let you know.

Financial Planning

By now you've got an idea of how much it costs to care for your new family member, and you're either pleasantly surprised or in a panic. If it's the former, pat yourself on the back and consider saving your extra pennies in a university fund for your child (an independent financial advisor can help you explore your options).

If you're in the panic category, take a deep breath and try to pinpoint the problem. Are the extra expenses coming from baby gadgetry and other non-essential purchases, or from necessities like nappies and wipes? A budget is really important in assessing the family finances now, so if you didn't create one during pregnancy, now is the time to start. There are places to cut back if you look for them.

Finally, if you find yourself hopelessly in debt, no matter how you look at the situation, you need to see a reputable debt counsellor or independent financial advisor to get back on your financial footing. See Chapter 3 for more tips on money management.

The Next Time Around

The first birthday is usually about the time when everyone starts asking about a brother or sister for your 'big' kid. When you're finished rolling your eyes and laughing, you start to actually give it some serious consideration. Are you ready to do it all over again?

Beyond physical readiness, how will you know? Suddenly, the sight of another woman in her ninth month brings about warm memories instead of enormous relief that it's someone else and not you, and you seem to have all but forgotten the perils of pregnancy and pain of childbirth.

If you're sold on a family with kids close enough in age to play and go to the same school together, you may be ready to start . Ggive your body time to recover so that you don't cheat yourself and your next child out of a healthy pregnancy. A two-year breather from birth to birth is ideal.

Losing any excess pounds before starting again will make it easier for you to get through and beyond the next pregnancy. And take the same pre-pregnancy precautions with folic acid supplements.

Just for Dads

Are you waiting for things to get back to normal? Stop right there. This is the new normal – take nothing for granted, be ready to change plans at a moment's notice, and learn to multitask. In other words, if you're a creature of habit and routine, you'll need to adjust your way of looking at the world.

The Night Shift

If you work a regular day job and then come home to play with and care for baby, it's easy to start burning the candle at both ends. You stay up later and later after baby's bedtime, to get things done or just unwind, and end up only getting a few hours of sleep on the clock before she's up for another feed. It's bad for your health and your sanity, so split the night shift with mum so you're at least getting all your sleep half the time.

Making Adjustments

Life as a father is full of compromise. The library you had started is now a playroom, and the motorcycle you've been lusting after has been shelved (even with a sidecar, it just wouldn't be the same). You plan to spend your weekend watching the World Cup, but reality strikes and you end up doing laps around the house with an ill, fretting baby instead. Yet instead of envying your childless friends who are at home doing what they want, you look at your child and wish you could take the hurt away and do it for her instead. Congratulations – you are a father.

Appendix A

Birth Plan Checklist

Consider starting your birth plan with a short note to both your doctor or midwife and the nursing staff who will be caring for you during labour and delivery. Explain your general wishes for a healthy and safe delivery, for joint decision-making should medical interventions be required, and for open communication throughout the process.

Read Chapter 15 to learn more about birth plans. Then use this checklist as a guide to assembling the basics.

1. Where will the birth take place?
   - ❑ Hospital
   - ❑ Birth centre
   - ❑ Home
   - ❑ Other: _____

2. Who will be there for labour support?
   - ❑ Husband or partner
   - ❑ Birth partner
   - ❑ Friend
   - ❑ Family member

3. Will any room modifications or equipment be required to increase your comfort mentally and physically?
   - ❑ Objects from home (e.g. pictures, blanket, pillow)
   - ❑ Lighting adjustments
   - ❑ Music
   - ❑ Video or photos of birth
   - ❑ Other: _____

4. Any special requests for labour prep procedures?
   - ❑ Forego enema
   - ❑ Self-administer enema
   - ❑ Forego shaving
   - ❑ Shave self
   - ❑ Heparin lock instead of routine IV line
   - ❑ Other: _____

5. Eating and drinking during labour?
   ❏ Want access to a light snack
   ❏ Want access to water, sports drink or other appropriate beverage
   ❏ Want ice cubes
   ❏ Other: _____

6. Do you want pain medication?
   ❏ Analgesic (e.g. Stadol, Demerol, Nubain)
   ❏ Epidural (if so, is timing an issue?)
   ❏ Other: _____

7. What non-pharmaceutical pain relief equipment might you want access to?
   ❏ Hydrotherapy (i.e. shower, whirlpool)
   ❏ Warm compresses
   ❏ Birth ball
   ❏ Other: _____

8. What interventions would you like to avoid unless deemed a medical necessity by your doctor during labour? Specify your preferred alternatives.
   ❏ Episiotomy
   ❏ Forceps
   ❏ Internal foetal monitoring
   ❏ Pitocin (oxytocin)
   ❏ Other: _____

9. What would you like your first face-to-face with baby to be like?
   ❏ Hold back on all non-essential treatment, evaluation and tests for a specified time.
   ❏ If immediate tests and evaluation are necessary, you, your partner or another support person will accompany baby.
   ❏ Want to nurse immediately following birth.
   ❏ Would like family members to meet baby immediately following birth.
   ❏ Other: _____

10. If a Caesarean birth is required, what is important to you and your partner?
    ❑ Type of anaesthesia (e.g. general vs. spinal block)
    ❑ Having partner or another support person present
    ❑ Spending time with baby immediately following procedure
    ❑ Bonding with baby in the recovery room
    ❑ Type of postoperative pain relief and nursing considerations
    ❑ Other: _____

11. Do you have a preference for who cuts the cord and when the cut is performed?
    ❑ Mum
    ❑ Dad
    ❑ Doctor or midwife
    ❑ Delay until cord stops pulsing.
    ❑ Cord blood will be banked. Cut per banking guidelines.
    ❑ Cut at doctor's discretion.
    ❑ Other: _____

12. What kind of postpartum care will you and baby have at the hospital?
    ❑ Baby will stay with mum.
    ❑ Baby will sleep in the nursery at night.
    ❑ Baby will breast-feed.
    ❑ Baby will bottle-feed.
    ❑ Baby will not be fed any supplemental formula and/or glucose water unless medically indicated.
    ❑ Baby will not be given a dummy.
    ❑ Other: _____

13. Considerations for after discharge.
    ❑ Support and short-term care for siblings
    ❑ Support if you've had a Caesarean
    ❑ Maternity leave
    ❑ Other: _____

Estimated Due Date Table

This chart lists due dates by month. Find the month and date on which your last menstrual period began, then look below that line to see what your estimated due date is.

If your last period was...	1/1	2/1	3/1	4/1	5/1	6/1	7/1	8/1
Then your EDD is...	8/10	9/10	10/10	11/10	12/10	13/10	14/10	15/10
If your last period was...	9/1	10/1	11/1	12/1	13/1	14/1	15/1	16/1
Then your EDD is...	16/10	17/10	18/10	19/10	20/10	21/10	22/10	23/10
If your last period was...	17/1	18/1	19/1	20/1	21/1	22/1	23/1	24/1
Then your EDD is...	24/10	25/10	26/10	27/10	28/10	29/10	30/10	31/10
If your last period was...	25/1	26/1	27/1	28/1	29/1	30/1	31/1	
Then your EDD is...	1/11	2/11	3/11	4/11	5/11	6/11	7/11	
If your last period was...	1/2	2/2	3/2	4/2	5/2	6/2	7/2	8/2
Then your EDD is...	8/11	9/11	10/11	11/11	12/11	13/11	14/11	15/11
If your last period was...	9/2	10/2	11/2	12/2	13/2	14/2	15/2	16/2
Then your EDD is...	16/11	17/11	18/11	19/11	20/11	21/11	22/11	23/11
If your last period was...	17/2	18/2	19/2	20/2	21/2	22/2	23/2	24/2
Then your EDD is...	24/11	25/11	26/11	27/11	28/11	29/11	30/11	1/12
If your last period was...	25/2	26/2	27/2	28/2				
Then your EDD is...	2/12	3/12	4/12	5/12				
If your last period was...	1/3	2/3	3/3	4/3	5/3	6/3	7/3	8/3
Then your EDD is...	6/12	7/12	8/12	9/12	10/12	11/12	12/12	13/12
If your last period was...	9/3	10/3	11/3	12/3	13/3	14/3	15/3	16/3
Then your EDD is...	14/12	15/12	16/12	17/12	18/12	19/12	20/12	21/12
If your last period was...	17/3	18/3	19/3	20/3	21/3	22/3	23/3	24/3
Then your EDD is...	22/12	23/12	24/12	25/12	26/12	27/12	28/12	29/12
If your last period was...	25/3	26/3	27/3	28/3	29/3	30/3	31/3	
Then your EDD is...	30/12	31/12	1/1	2/1	3/1	4/1	5/1	
If your last period was...	1/4	2/4	3/4	4/4	5/4	6/4	7/4	8/4
Then your EDD is...	6/1	7/1	8/1	9/1	10/1	11/1	12/1	13/1
If your last period was...	9/4	10/4	11/4	12/4	13/4	14/4	15/4	16/4
Then your EDD is...	14/1	15/1	16/1	17/1	18/1	19/1	20/1	21/1
If your last period was...	17/4	18/4	19/4	20/4	21/4	22/4	23/4	24/4
Then your EDD is...	22/1	23/1	24/1	25/1	26/1	27/1	28/1	29/1
If your last period was...	25/4	26/4	27/4	28/4	29/4	30/4		
Then your EDD is...	30/1	31/1	1/2	2/2	3/2	4/2		
If your last period was...	1/5	2/5	3/5	4/5	5/5	6/5	7/5	8/5

Then your EDD is...	5/2	6/2	7/2	8/2	9/2	10/2	11/2	12/2

If your last period was...	9/5	10/5	11/5	12/5	13/5	14/5	15/5	16/5
Then your EDD is...	13/2	14/2	15/2	16/2	17/2	18/2	19/2	20/2

If your last period was...	17/5	18/5	19/5	20/5	21/5	22/5	23/5	24/5
Then your EDD is...	21/2	22/2	23/2	24/2	25/2	26/2	27/2	28/2

If your last period was...	25/2	26/5	27/5	28/5	29/5	30/5	31/5	
Then your EDD is...	1/3	2/3	3/3	4/3	5/3	6/3	7/3	

If your last period was...	1/6	2/6	3/6	4/6	5/6	6/6	7/6	8/6
Then your EDD is...	8/3	9/3	10/3	11/3	12/3	13/3	14/3	15/3

If your last period was...	9/6	10/6	11/6	12/6	13/6	14/6	15/6	16/6
Then your EDD is...	16/3	17/3	18/3	19/3	20/3	21/3	22/3	23/3

If your last period was...	17/6	18/6	19/6	20/6	21/6	22/6	23/6	24/6
Then your EDD is...	24/3	25/3	26/3	27/3	28/3	29/3	30/3	31/3

If your last period was...	25/6	26/6	27/6	28/6	29/6	30/6		
Then your EDD is...	1/4	2/4	3/4	4/4	5/4	6/4		

If your last period was...	1/7	2/7	7/3	4/7	5/7	6/7	7/7	8/7
Then your EDD is...	7/4	8/4	9/4	10/4	11/4	12/4	13/4	14/4

If your last period was...	9/7	10/7	11/7	12/7	13/7	14/7	15/7	16/7
Then your EDD is...	15/4	16/4	17/4	18/4	19/4	20/4	21/4	22/4

If your last period was...	17/7	18/7	19/7	20/7	21/7	22/7	23/7	24/7
Then your EDD is...	23/4	24/4	25/4	26/4	27/4	28/4	29/4	30/4

If your last period was...	25/7	26/7	27/7	28/7	29/7	30/7	31/7	
Then your EDD is...	1/5	2/5	3/5	4/5	5/5	6/5	7/5	

If your last period was...	1/8	2/8	3/8	4/8	5/8	6/8	7/8	8/8
Then your EDD is...	8/5	9/5	10/5	11/5	12/5	13/5	14/5	15/5

If your last period was...	9/8	10/8	11/8	12/8	13/8	14/8	15/8	16/8
Then your EDD is...	16/5	17/5	18/5	19/5	20/5	21/5	22/5	23/5

If your last period was...	17/8	18/8	19/8	20/8	21/8	22/8	23/8	24/8
Then your EDD is...	24/5	25/5	26/5	27/5	28/5	29/5	30/5	31/5

If your last period was...	25/8	26/8	27/8	28/8	29/8	30/8	31/8	
Then your EDD is...	1/6	2/6	3/6	4/6	5/6	6/6	7/6	

If your last period was...	1/9	2/9	3/9	4/9	5/9	6/9	7/9	8/9
Then your EDD is...	8/6	9/6	10/6	11/6	12/6	13/6	14/6	15/6

| If your last period was... | 9/9 | 10/9 | 11/9 | 12/9 | 13/9 | 14/9 | 15/9 | 16/9 |
| Then your EDD is... | 16/6 | 17/6 | 18/6 | 19/6 | 20/6 | 21/6 | 22/6 | 23/6 |

| If your last period was... | 17/9 | 18/9 | 19/9 | 20/9 | 21/9 | 22/9 | 23/9 | 24/9 |
| Then your EDD is... | 24/6 | 25/6 | 26/6 | 27/6 | 28/6 | 29/6 | 30/6 | 1/7 |

| If your last period was... | 25/9 | 26/9 | 27/9 | 28/9 | 29/9 | 30/9 | | |
| Then your EDD is... | 2/7 | 3/7 | 4/7 | 5/7 | 6/7 | 7/7 | | |

| If your last period was... | 1/10 | 2/10 | 3/10 | 4/10 | 5/10 | 6/10 | 7/10 | 8/10 |
| Then your EDD is... | 8/7 | 9/7 | 10/7 | 11/7 | 12/7 | 13/7 | 14/7 | 15/7 |

| If your last period was... | 9/10 | 10/10 | 11/10 | 12/10 | 13/10 | 14/10 | 15/10 | 16/10 |
| Then your EDD is... | 16/7 | 17/7 | 18/7 | 19/7 | 20/7 | 21/7 | 22/7 | 23/7 |

| If your last period was... | 17/10 | 18/10 | 19/10 | 20/10 | 21/10 | 22/10 | 23/10 | 24/10 |
| Then your EDD is... | 24/7 | 25/7 | 26/7 | 27/7 | 28/7 | 29/7 | 30/7 | 31/7 |

| If your last period was... | 25/10 | 26/10 | 27/10 | 28/10 | 29/10 | 30/10 | 31/10 | |
| Then your EDD is... | 1/8 | 2.8 | 3/8 | 4/8 | 5/8 | 6/8 | 7/8 | |

| If your last period was... | 1/11 | 2/11 | 3/11 | 4/11 | 5/11 | 6/11 | 7/11 | 8/11 |
| Then your EDD is... | 8/8 | 9/8 | 10/8 | 11/8 | 12/8 | 13/8 | 14/8 | 15/8 |

| If your last period was... | 9/11 | 10/11 | 11/11 | 12/11 | 13/11 | 14/11 | 15/11 | 16/11 |
| Then your EDD is... | 16/8 | 17/8 | 18/8 | 19/8 | 20/8 | 21/8 | 22/8 | 23/8 |

| If your last period was... | 17/11 | 18/11 | 19/11 | 20/11 | 21/11 | 22/11 | 23/11 | 24/11 |
| Then your EDD is... | 24/8 | 25/8 | 26/8 | 27/8 | 28/8 | 29/8 | 30/8 | 31/8 |

| If your last period was... | 25/11 | 26/11 | 27/11 | 28/11 | 29/11 | 30/11 | | |
| Then your EDD is... | 1/9 | 2/9 | 3/9 | 4/9 | 5/9 | 6/9 | | |

| If your last period was... | 1/12 | 2/12 | 3/12 | 4/12 | 5/12 | 6/12 | 7/12 | 8/12 |
| Then your EDD is... | 7/9 | 8/9 | 9/9 | 10/9 | 11/9 | 12/9 | 13/9 | 14/9 |

| If your last period was... | 9/12 | 10/12 | 11/12 | 12/12 | 13/12 | 14/12 | 15/12 | 16/12 |
| Then your EDD is... | 15/9 | 16/9 | 17/9 | 18/9 | 19/9 | 20/9 | 21/9 | 22/9 |

| If your last period was... | 17/12 | 18/12 | 19/12 | 20/12 | 21/12 | 22/12 | 23/12 | 24/12 |
| Then your EDD is... | 23/9 | 24/9 | 25/9 | 26/9 | 27/9 | 28/9 | 29/9 | 30/9 |

| If your last period was... | 25/12 | 26/12 | 27/12 | 28/12 | 29/12 | 30/12 | 31/12 | |
| Then your EDD is... | 1/10 | 2/10 | 3/10 | 4/10 | 5/10 | 6/10 | 7/10 | |

A ppendix C

The Practical Side
of Pregnancy –
A Nine-Month Checklist

Your health-care provider will keep you abreast of what medical steps you should be taking throughout your pregnancy, but there are plenty of practical matters you and your partner will need to address that aren't covered by doctor's orders. This month-by-month checklist provides a handy reference list to make sure you've covered the basics. Rearrange the timeline to your own schedule and pregnancy, if needed, and turn to the referenced chapters for further details and tips on each item.

Month 1

❑ Evaluate your doctor or group practice and decide if it's right for you and your pregnancy. (Chapter 1)
❑ Get up to speed on your health insurance coverage for prenatal visits, delivery and the care of your child. (Chapter 3)
❑ If you smoke or drink, stop now. (Chapter 1)
❑ Discuss any possible on-the-job hazards with your doctor. (Chapter 9)

Month 2

❑ Start developing a maternity wardrobe. (Chapter 4)
❑ Take inventory of what baby or maternity items you will 'inherit' from friends and family. (Chapter 4)
❑ Share the good news with your other kids. (Chapter 11)
❑ Sit down with your partner and start working out a post-baby budget. (Chapter 3)

Month 3

❑ Inform your employer. (Chapters 6 and 9)
❑ Get details on your maternity benefits. (Chapter 9)
❑ Look into a prenatal exercise class. (Chapter 8)
❑ Decide where the baby's room or space will be. (Chapter 3)
❑ Make sleep a priority; set a new early bedtime and stick to it. (Chapter 10)

Month 4

❑ Treat yourself and your kids to a special day out. (Chapters 11 and 12)
❑ Compare and decide on cloth versus disposable nappies. (Chapter 16)
❑ Find out how and when to add your new baby to your insurance coverage. (Chapter 3)
❑ If you don't have one, shop for a cot that meets current safety standards. (Chapter 3)
❑ Do some basic babyproofing. (Chapter 3)

Month 5

❑ Plan a special night out with your partner. (Chapter 12)
❑ Perform a pre-baby car check. (Chapter 3)
  · Ensure that your vehicle is child-seat-friendly.
  · Purchase a rear-facing infant seat for your child.
  · Try your hand at properly installing it in your vehicle.
❑ Explore child-care options for your new baby. (Chapters 9 and 21)

Month 6

❑ Take a day off and pamper yourself. (Chapter 12)
❑ Start putting together your birth plan. (Chapter 15)
❑ Think about who you want in the delivery room. (Chapter 15)
❑ Contemplate the breast versus bottle decision. (Chapter 19)
❑ Discuss your maternity-leave plans with your employer. (Chapter 9)

Month 7

❑ Make a date with yourself to relax, read or just catch up on sleep. (Chapter 12)
❑ Sign up for childbirth classes. (Chapter 14)
❑ Sign your child up for sibling classes. (Chapters 11 and 14)

❑ Set up an appointment to discuss your birth plan with your health-care provider. (Chapter 15)

❑ Arrange for care for your other children during your hospital stay. (Chapter 17)

Month 8

❑ Take five and de-stress; it's good for you and baby. (Chapter 4)

❑ Prepare baby's room or sleep space. (Chapter 3)

❑ Lay out your baby essentials. (Chapter 16)

❑ Start wrapping up projects at work. (Chapter 9)

❑ Finalize your child care plans for after-maternity leave. (Chapters 9 and 21)

Month 9

❑ Make sure that your other children's teachers and care providers are aware of your impending hospital stay. (Chapter 17)

❑ Pack your bag and compile a call list for your partner. (Chapter 17)

❑ Line up postpartum assistance. (Chapter 17)

❑ Stock up the freezer with quick meals, or recruit postpartum kitchen help. (Chapter 17)

❑ Make a plan and a back-up plan for getting to the hospital. (Chapter 17)

❑ Put your feet up, relax and take a deep breath – the rest is up to baby!

V

Vacuum extraction, 241
Vaginal birth after cesarean
(VBAC), 131–45, 182, 240
Vaginal bleeding, 102, 120, 156,
157, 161, 164–73, 167, 170
Vaginal delivery
after cesarean sections, 131–45,
182
for breech births, 201–24
moment of, 230–49
for multiple births, 86
Vaginal discharge, 19, 24, 47, 167,
169, 171, 177
Vaginal infections, 168
Vaginal secretions, 18–19
Vanishing twin syndrome, 86
Varicella infection, 61, 99
Varicose veins, 119

Vehicle safety, 33–34, 147
Vernix caseosa, 119
Vertex position, 86, 198
Videotaping, 189, 193
Vision problems, 24, 102, 146, 166,
200, 201
Vitamins, 7–9, 23, 27, 284
Vomiting. See Morning sickness

W

Water, drinking, 83, 97, 257, 267,
284
Water retention, 146, 200
'Waters breaking', 212
Weight gain
breakdown of, 70–71
excessive weight gain, 146
first trimester, 46, 69
individuality of, 73

second trimester, 96
slowdown in, 199, 211
stretch marks, 119–36
sudden weight gain, 166
third trimester, 199, 211
Weight lifting, 107
Weight loss
of baby, 268
of mother, 160, 258, 282, 290
Wine, 6–7
Womb. See Uterus
Work issues, 105–32, 218, 246,
286–12

X, Y, Z

X-rays, 107, 107
Yolk sac, 17
Zygote, 16